Energy

the

Essence

of

Environmental

Health

Alan R. Vinitsky, M.D.   Natalie Golos

PRELUDE

Stress STRESS STRESS!

Chaos! Our contemporary world is littered with the excess affects of fast, faster, fastest, discord, electronics, air pollution, terrorism, violence, fear, illness and more! **How can you and your family survive the perils of this stressful existence?**

Natalie Golos and Alan Vinitsky provide the answer in **Energy – the Essence of Environmental Health** — engaging, easy-to-follow and injected with humor. Their life stories form the foundation for discovering the secret to achieving Optimal Health. Often overlooked by health care practitioners, the Autonomic Nervous System (ANS) silently regulates all bodily functions. Symptoms of illness often present when the ANS attempts to correct itself. Chronic illness results when the ANS remains unstable. The model of the **Accordion Reserve©** represents the fluctuating effects of the ANS.

How do you recognize your ANS? Is Fatigue interfering with your lifestyle? Are you scared speechless? Are moody blues bringing you down? Is your heart thumping with minimal provocation? Do you get short winded during trivial exertion? Is the closest lavatory just not close enough? Listen to your erratic vibrational rhythms! That's your ANS chattering.

Follow along as the authors guide you on the path to optimal sleep, exercise, nutrition and relationships with yourself, others, your environment and your Guiding Force. Learn to breathe correctly, meditate, relax and discover. The basis for success is your own Body Awareness – a Flashback to Infancy. The result is a balanced ANS.

Apply these lessons to improved parenting, treating developmental disorders, hyperactivity, autistic spectrum and mood disorders. Anticipate and avert chronic diseases such as diabetes, heart ailments and environmentally triggered illnesses before they start.

First published by AuthorHouse 09/14/04

ISBN: 1-4184-7019-8 (e)
ISBN: 1-4184-3347-0 (sc)
ISBN: 1-4184-3349-7 (dj)

Library of Congress Control Number: 2003098487

Printed in the United States of America
Bloomington, Indiana

This book is printed on acid-free paper.

Authors' Notes

Note that the word "he" is used throughout the book as shorthand for "he" and "she" and is not meant to imply gender discrimination, male superiority or the authors' laziness.

Energy – the Essence of Environmental Health is not a substitute for proper medical diagnosis and treatment. Consult a competent professional for solutions to your specific concerns.

LIBRARY OF CONGRESS CATALOGING-IN-PUBLICATION DATA:
Golos, Natalie.

Energy – the Essence of Environmental Health / Natalie Golos and Alan R. Vinitsky, M.D.

1. Environmental health. 2. Energy. 3. Spiritual Healing. 4. Meditation/Relaxation Healing.
5. Autonomic nervous system. 6. Lessons from Theron Randolph, M.D.
7. Pediatric behavior modification. 8. Deconditioning violence.
I. Vinitsky, Alan R. II. Title.

ACKNOWLEDGMENTS

The materials gathered for this work have been compiled from the rich and varied experiences of many Environmental Medicine Practitioners, Energy Therapists, and more significantly, countless individuals who have learned to cope with their illness.

A special thanks to patients who allowed us to demonstrate how they used our guidelines to develop their own unique health program.

We are grateful to Larry Plumlee, M.D. for his insightful suggestions and Alyce Ortuzar and John Michael Wilhere for editing the food lists.

Words cannot express our indebtedness and appreciation to three special individuals:

James Cox, Dr. theol. (pastoral counselor), who initiated our study of therapeutic/spiritual energy fields and who gave valuable advice and suggestions on every phase of stress management that is discussed in this work.

Marcia Marks, a devoted volunteer activist who quietly behind the scenes has diligently pursued social changes at the community, state and national levels, as she carried the banner for prevention of illness caused by tobacco, pesticides and radiation, etc.

Allan Jablon, our final editor, whose valuable advice and suggestions often changed our approach of presentation. His knowledge in applied physics and electrical engineering has had a greater impact than even he can imagine.

And, to both our families, who know in their hearts that their encouragement, support and love have inspired us to fulfill our dream.

We are especially blessed to have two special family members in our prayers:

I, Natalie, wish to pay tribute to my sister Frances Golos Golbitz, co-author of my previous books. No one, not even Fran, can possibly understand that without her I would never have become an author. In our first books, she found words to express my thoughts as I struggled to extract them from my encephalopathic brain. Thank you Fran, I love you.

Alan's wife Ruth is also very special to me because she initially "adopted me" into the Vinitsky family. Through her kindness she and their children – Emily, Seth and Ariel – have filled a personal void because my closely-knit family is separated geographically.

I, Alan, thank my beautiful wife Ruth who has stood beside me and with me during our worst nightmares of the past few years. Especially she has endured more stress than I can imagine, and it is no secret to everyone else we know and love, that she is my special treasure. I will always love her.

DEDICATION
in
MEMORIAM

To Theron Randolph, M.D. who hypothesized that successful treatment of chemical susceptibility (now called Environmentally Triggered Illness – ETI) correlated directly with sound education that is as important as the doctor's contribution.

♪♪♪♪♪

After hearing my paper on patient education at the Denver 1974 Eighth Advanced Seminar of the American Academy of Environmental Medicine, Randolph solicited a promise from me to continue to spread his word to patients, doctors and the public at large, even after his death.[1]

Alan has joined forces with me to help fulfill that promise to Dr. Randolph.

♪♪♪♪♪

Natalie Golos   *Alan R. Vinitsky*

---

[1] *Energy – the Essence of Environmental Health* will be a vehicle to raise funds to preserve and maintain the Randolph Library at the Southwest College of Naturopathic Medicine and Health Sciences.

CONTENTS

FOREWORD

♫♫♫♫♫

Energy – the Essence of Environmental Health is a tribute to Dr. Theron Randolph, father of Environmental Medicine. In honor of his memory, we created a framework that incorporates time-tested skills, dedication and caring that Dr. Randolph represented.

Dr. Theron Randolph was the Master Medical Listener. Many tributes were written in his honor on the occasion of his passing.* Dr. Ken Gerdes remembers Dr. Randolph as the consummate physician. By permission we quote Dr. Gerdes because his tribute clearly identifies Dr. Randoph's excellence:

"As a student physician working for Dr. Randolph, I heard the story of how he 'broke the chemical problem.' His patient was a physician's wife from Michigan with severe migraines and multiple other symptoms. Her case is described on pages 12-15 of Randolph's book, *Human Ecology and Susceptibility to the Chemical Environment*.[1] What does not appear in the case report is the interaction between patient and physician.

"She had been to a great many physicians. None had been able to help her. Dr. Randolph did not know if he could help her either. So he agreed with her that he would LISTEN to what she could tell him of what was happening to her. He would not charge for his listening, but he hoped to learn something from her story which might be useful for other patients.

"So he listened for more than a year of appointments, more than 50 pages of single-spaced typewritten notes. Then there came a day when he could sit down with her and go over all of those notes. Dr. Randolph told me, 'I read about 2/3 of the way through and suddenly I could see that every time she had the headaches she had been exposed to petrochemicals. Then it was easy to set up a test to prove it.'

Environmental Physician, 1996, Fall Issue. You can obtain a memorial copy of these tributes by contacting Central Office, American Academy of Environmental Medicine, 7701 East Kellogg, Suite 625, Wichita, KS 67207. Telephone 316-684-5500, fax 316-684-5709, e-mail http://www.aaem.com/.

"And more than 40 years later, a very large number of physicians who appear NOT to listen to their patients still dispute the observations Dr. Randolph made."

THE ECOLOGIC-ORIENTED HISTORY

In the dramatic case above, you can see that Dr. Randolph 1) took time to <u>listen</u>, and in so doing, he noted 2) <u>patterns and nature of exposure</u> and 3) <u>onset of symptoms</u>. Linking symptoms with patterns of exposures came to be known as "THE ECOLOGIC-ORIENTED HISTORY" (EOH) – the common thread that binds all who practice Randolph's concepts.

In spite of the adherence to the EOH practice of Environmental Medicine (EM), practitioners of EM demonstrate their uniqueness by following Randolph's openness to new ideas. Even as we notice the similarities of national and international EM practices, we are always acutely aware of their differences.

Some of our philosophy is new but is grounded in the experience, teaching and legacy of Dr. Randolph. In the course of your reading *Energy – the Essence of Environmental Health*, you will be introduced to some of the other giants in the field – Dr. William Rea, Dr. Doris Rapp and others we acknowledge throughout the book. These practitioners and other students of Dr. Randolph have advanced his fundamental understanding of Environmental Medicine.

In accepting his approach of the EOH,[2] the early Environmental Practitioners called themselves "Clinical Ecologists." They used the word "ecology" to describe the study of an organism's behavior in relation to its environment.

Unfortunately, the expression "Clinical Ecology" acquired a negative connotation because critics of the field claimed that there was "insufficient science" to justify its utility.

In an effort to escape criticism, "Clinical Ecology" was renamed "Environmental Medicine." The principles of dedication to the original EOH remain. Yet the name change has not stilled the criticism.

Practitioners of EM often encounter a similar lack of respect. Blanket criticisms without basis are still made by some who describe "Environmental Physicians" as practicing with techniques and tests that are out of the standard of medical care. And these criticisms still receive significant media exposure.

Whatever the terminology, the subject matter has always appealed to me. I included ecology in my undergraduate zoology honors studies. My medical practice and life-long journey are natural extensions of my early endeavors in and observation of human nature and communications – verbal and non-verbal.

This book is about listening, observing and learning, just as Dr. Randolph taught us. Its appeal is for anyone who seeks information about "Clinical Ecology" or EM and what they offer you as a practitioner, patient or health-minded individual.

We seek to bridge differences, rather than divide and criticize. In fact, our model, the Accordion Reserve©, emphasizes what we believe: the EOH is rooted in the sound medical tradition of careful and thorough history taking, from which reasonable hypotheses can be suggested and tested. The complexities of that history often make researching the hypotheses difficult. Yet, that does not invalidate the history. We hope that the Accordion Reserve© offers support to the concept that "the absence of proof is not proof of absence."[3]

Dr. Randolph practiced medicine by treating patients with humanity, caring and respect, while applying sound medical principles that are founded in science. I never had the privilege of studying personally with Dr. Randolph, but I feel that I have, because I have benefited from those he taught.

Natalie personally worked with Dr. Randolph as patient and educator. Natalie encouraged me to attend my first meetings sponsored by the American Academy of Environmental Medicine (AAEM). I was "kicking all the way" because I didn't believe I would have anything to gain by attending. I am grateful to her and the teachers at those meetings, who have helped me find my way. Natalie and the other pioneers link us to Dr. Randolph, keeping his traditions alive and vibrant.

Dr. Randolph once wrote: "Patients must be educated in both the philosophy and distinctive features of this type of medicine, as well as in the details of applying it."[4] To this end we present our book *Energy – the Essence of Environmental Health*.

Here are some suggestions on how to use *Energy – the Essence of Environmental Health* to best advantage:

* SCAN THE TABLE OF CONTENTS. In keeping with the wisdom of Dr. Randolph we divided the Contents into seven parts. Indispensable are the first two parts, in which we detail the philosophy of our work. Parts III through VII provide applications, incorporating our personal experiences as examples, for you to use as guidelines to develop your own program.

* PAY ATTENTION TO THE CHAPTER ORDER. Recognize the theme of an EOH.

* READ THE CHAPTER TITLES. Discover the power of Listening to your Body and its environment. In this context, "listening" means "feeling, sensing, focusing or hearing with your ears." In other words, you are encouraged to take a sensory inventory of your body.

* READ NATALIE AND ALAN'S STORIES. Observe how helpful it was for us to follow Randolph's teaching. Pay special attention to the linkage between onset of symptoms and exposures. Follow our guidelines to do the same for yourself.

* READ THE CHAPTERS. Learn to associate your feelings, sensations and reactions to your Body Awareness.
    * Experience the lessons, beginning in Part III.
    * Periodically return to Part II Chapters to understand your healing experiences.

* SEARCH FOR YOUR PERSONAL PATTERNS. Recall Dr. Randolph's groundbreaking case and our stories.

* EXPLORE AND ENGAGE YOUR INTUITION. Emulate but do not copy our experiences.

* LISTEN FOR THE MUSICAL THEME. Feel and heal as you play "the Accordion Reserve©."

Experience how the Accordion Reserve© evolved into a model that bridges and unites multiple approaches to health care.

In *Energy – the Essence of Environmental Health* we compile and assimilate information gathered from seminars, books and personal experiences. We adapted these experiences to our particular field and interest of ENVIRONMENTAL MEDICINE. Intuitively we identified programs, actions and behaviors that others have recognized before us.

Unique to our shared experiences was our awareness that our environment is simultaneously within us and around us. The Accordion Reserve© model was born from this recognition. In that moment of Enlightenment, our Awakening, we experienced the unity of Environment and Mind/body/soul/spirit.

Alan R. Vinitsky

---

[1] Randolph TG. 1962. *Human Ecology and Susceptibility to the Chemical Environment.* Charles C Thomas, Publisher, Springfield, IL.

[2] AAEM - copyrighted versions that help professionals follow the EOH. See Appendix D.

[3] Hoffmeier J. "Who was Moses?" *Time Magazine.* December 14, 1998, p. 82.

[4] Randolph, T. 1979, revised 1988. Foreword to *Coping with Your Allergies,* Golos N, Golbitz F. Simon & Schuster, NY.

PREFACE

Have you visited doctor after doctor, unsuccessfully seeking answers to your questions in order to get yourself well?

Do you avoid going to a mainstream medical doctor?
Do you avoid going to an "alternative" practitioner?
Does your conventional health care practitioner reject your alternative provider's opinion and *vice versa*?

Why do conventional physicians reject opinions of board-certified physicians who practice Environmental Medicine?

Does your conventional physician reject your requests for referral to a board-certified specialist who also practices Environmental Medicine?

Does your insurance company reject your request for referral to a board-certified specialist who also practices Environmental Medicine?

Then you're part of a 50-year-old Medical Controversy! What is the basis for this Medical Controversy?

Where does Belief begin and Science end? Where does Science begin and Belief end? Would you agree that these questions are the basis for one of Life's enduring Mysteries?

When we contemplate healing — Is it a concern of Science? Of Spirit? Or both?

We hope that *Energy – the Essence of Environmental Health* will stimulate a thought-provoking debate that:

♪ Unearths this Controversy and Mystery
♪ Provides a unique model that links mind and body, soul and spirit, health and healing to Energy and the power of the Autonomic Nervous System

♫ Affords the medical and spiritual communities with a working hypothesis to stimulate joint research that could resolve this Controversy and the Mystery

Energy – the Essence of Environmental Health also

♫ Uses self-revealing human interest examples to:
  ♫ Teach you how to maintain and achieve optimal health
  ♫ Provide step-by-step procedures to gain Awareness of your Personal Energy
  ♫ Instruct you in expanding your Personal Energy
  ♫ Guide you in learning practical environmental safeguards to maintain or restore your health
  ♫ Teach you how to balance your Autonomic Nervous System

Energy – the Essence of Environmental Health presents the **Accordion Reserve**©, the authors' working model for attaining your optimal health level in the polluted environment and over-stressed lifestyle of the 21st Century. In light of the aftermath from September 11, 2001, our model has an even greater impact for dealing with the universal tragedy of death and destruction – especially for the heroes who toiled in the devastation of the polluted environment.

OUR SYMBOL

The model of the **Accordion Reserve**© presents a visual/manual teaching tool to simplify the message of the human body's Energy Reserve. Read this book to learn why the authors chose the Accordion as the best visual, tangible and audible representation of the human body. In our book we refer to a human being as a unified Thinking Mind, Physical Body, Soul and Spirit. Learn to use the model to develop your own health plan as unique as your DNA and fingerprints. As you heal you will discover your own unity – Mind/body/soul/spirit.

The Reserve represents your fluctuating Energy/Stress Level (your body's level of tolerance).

xx

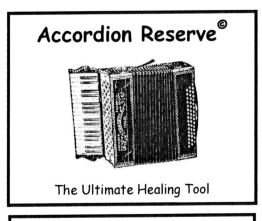

| Figure P-1. The Accordion Reserve©. |

MUSICAL ANALOGY

Our musical analogy illustrates the dynamic effects of stress on your health. The continuous interplay of the accordion's handles and bellows over time represents the complex relationships of Environmental Stressors and Energy Stressors. Biologically, chemically, physically, mentally, emotionally, spiritually and interpersonally, the accordion expands and contracts, defining the extent of your Reserve.

The Accordion	Your Body
Right Keyboard Handle	Your Environment
Left Button Handle	Your Energy
Bellows	Your Lungs
Musical Frequencies	Your Energy Frequencies

Figure P-2. Accordion Analogy. The accordion represents your body's environment and energy.

The Accordion Reserve© concept also helps you learn to use your body as several types of musical instruments, as well as your own generator.

TEAM WORK

The authors' collaboration represents the melding of personal, professional and educational experiences in Environmental, Alternative, Naturopathic, Orthomolecular, Preventive, Traditional, Oriental, Native American and Mainstream Western Medicine as well as therapeutic and fitness techniques.

SUCCESS OF THE ACCORDION RESERVE©

♪♪♪♪

For the Chronically Ill I, Natalie, demonstrate how I used our combined techniques to recover from partial paralysis, toxic encephalopathy (brain damage caused by toxic chemicals), memory loss and severe environmentally triggered illness (ETI). My personal story will always be introduced by ♪♪♪♪ and will appear in this font.

♫♫♫♫♫

For the Relatively Healthy Thinking I was normal and healthy, I, Alan, demonstrate how I use the combined techniques to prevent a serious illness I now know was beginning to manifest in my body. My personal story will always be introduced by ♫♫♫♫♫ and appear in this font.

♫♫♫♫♫

RESTORING YOUR ENVIRONMENTAL HEALTH

Please join us as we travel on our musical journey to promote personal growth. Use our guidelines, your own past experiences and your own creativity to develop your own success.

In each chapter look for the expression **Accordion Reserve©** to highlight lessons that guide you. While it may seem redundant to repeat the phrase, we hope that through conditioning you will gain strength in developing your unique Environmental Health program.

PART I

Discoveries by Listening

LESSONS from DR. RANDOLPH

1
SERENDIPITY -
or <u>Was</u> It by Chance?

Prologue

Our story is one infinitesimal speck in time, yet we believe that, by the power of example, you may gain new insight from grasping life's opportunities.

From our very first meeting, there were more questions than answers. We raise them for you to ponder as you read the story of our evolving journey together.

Why did we meet? Was it Serendipity? - Or Coincidence? - Or Synchronicity?

Do people react to a Plan? Are they part of a Plan? Do they create their own Plan? Do they have Choice? Are they Pre-destined?

♪♪♪♪

One of my previous co-authors William Rea, M.D. was a guest lecturer at Shady Grove Adventist Hospital, so I attended the presentation. Alan peppered Dr. Rea with questions so probing that I couldn't avoid noticing. I invited Alan to attend meetings of the Mid-Atlantic Environmental Medicine Network, which he did, as I found out much later, quite reluctantly.

Alan attended a session of my teaching workshop for environmentally ill patients. I encouraged Alan to attend a strategy meeting at Marcia Marks[i] home. At that meeting, we discussed the topic "Violence Caused by Legal and Illegal

---

[i] Marks, Marcia. Advocate for Environmental Issues on the community level – for example, pesticides, smoking and radiation. See Appendix D.

3

Drugs." The information gathered was to have been presented to a physician on General Barry McCaffrey's staff.[i] The staff conference never occurred, but as "fate would have it," Alan had written an essay on violence and brought it to the strategy session. Marcia and I read the essay and were impressed with his literary style and medical knowledge. I was thinking about writing another book and asked Alan to join me.

♫♫♫♫♫

I always wanted to write a book. For me, Natalie's offer seemed like a dream come true.
♫♫♫♫♫

"LIFE IS FULL OF SURPRISES"

<u>*Surprises or Messages?*</u> Risky? Neither of us knew what was in store. Our meeting opened a window of opportunity for us to grow. We followed our instincts and embarked on an adventure of personal health and growth.

COMMON THREADS

Why our title — *Energy – the Essence of Environmental Health?*

Environmental Health (EH) is the most powerful of all our common threads. However, Energy is more than EH — Energy is the essence of every experience of every living organism.

<u>*Common Paths*</u> As we grew, we discovered so many similarities in our life paths. It seemed that we were destined to meet.

Destiny? Merging? Uniting? Energy joined? Is Creativity an endless play on the Messages of a Guiding Force? Are there any Limits to Discovery?

---

[i] McCaffrey, General Barry. Clinton Administration "Drug Czar."

Discovery is open to those who open their senses to the world around them.

♫♫♫♫♫

Alan's Discovery Before we started on the book, Natalie taught me her stress reduction techniques, using visualization to achieve a relaxed state, to recognize my sensations and feeling.

The next day during my usual hour run, I felt what I call my "Awakening." I was duplicating the previous night's experience. This was the sensation that always made me feel so energized after running. However, this time my energy was intensified by a spontaneous visualization of my head attached to an old-fashioned streetcar wire. Serendipity! We changed Natalie's expression "the Feeling" to the more descriptive "the Awakening."

♫♫♫♫♫

FABRIC

Listening Our personal stories are scattered throughout relevant chapters rather than in chronological order. Whenever we worked together, we listened to ourselves and to each other. We listened to our bodies and our meditative insights. Our merging energetic development became another common thread.

Backgrounds Our diverse personal interests followed similar paths – teaching patients and self-healing:
  * *Alan's philosophy of teaching his pediatric patients' parents, obese patients and sports injured patients.*
  * *Alan's personal fitness program.*
  * *Natalie's experience teaching Environmentally Triggered Illness (ETI) patients, their families, physicians and their staff.*
  * *Natalie's search for a cure.*

TEXTURE

<u>*Flashpoint of Controversy*</u> We are besieged by a never-ending battle — Chemical Industry *vs.* Environmentalists, Mainstream Medicine *vs.* Alternative Medicine, Media *vs.* Everyone, and many more such polarized positions. It is time for healing to begin.

<u>*Weaving Philosophies and Disciplines*</u> We blend Western medicine and dentistry, Oriental medicine, Environmental Medicine and Dentistry, complementary and alternative medicine, integrative medicine, vibrational medicine, naturopathy, chiropractic, physical fitness, stress reduction, visualization and spiritual healing.

SEAMS

We sew threads, fabric and texture into a symbolic working model that questions the Controversy dividing the healthcare community. We unravel Life's Mystery by illustrating the complex interaction of our existence – our Energy and our Environment. Is it necessary to have a scientific background to grasp what has baffled generations? – Is it science? Is it Spirit? Is it both?

FINISHED ENSEMBLE?

The Accordion Reserve© *is our discovery.* During our brainstorming sessions we realized we could not separate our minds from one another or our energies from one another. What began as a project to write a book became a new living experience of the power of the Accordion Reserve©, the power of "Awakening," the power of the aura and the power of human energy in friendship.

SUMMARY

What is it that unites people in various causes? Love of God? Love of a Guiding Force? Love of children? Love of causes? Love of Nature? Love of Music? Similar energies for a common purpose? " Is it by chance?"

2
NATALIE'S STORY
- Full Circle -
Health
/ Brush with Death /
Health Restored

♫♫♫♫♫

The Mystery of My Paralysis Many years ago, every fourth Wednesday I would awaken paralyzed on my left side. By the weekend, I regained use of my left arm and leg and was able to ride my bicycle again. Why did it occur every Wednesday? Why did it take longer to recover every fifth Wednesday?

Detective Work After months of checking patterns as taught by Dr. Randolph, Dr. Kailin and I could find nothing in my house that was unusual on Wednesday. Because I am a delayed reactor, my doctor finally decided to investigate what happened on Tuesday in my brand new all electric 25-story luxury apartment building, which, ironically, I had recently rented for health purposes.

Mystery Solved We discovered that for prevention purposes, every Tuesday exterminators sprayed garbage compactor chutes, five floors at a time. After five weeks they started over again. During the week they sprayed the tenth through the fifteenth floors (I lived on the twelfth), my paralysis lasted longer than the other four weeks.

THE POWER OF THOUGHTS

How I Turned a Negative into a Positive I kept reminding myself how lucky I was that from a list of unknown

7

allergists I had chosen Dr. Eloise Kailin as my doctor. She was probably the only local doctor who realized symptoms like mine were not imagined.

Environmentally triggered illness (ETI) is a physiologic abnormality. There is now substantial scientific evidence demonstrating effects of toxins on the central nervous system. Granted, people may also have psychological illnesses, separate or secondary to ETI. As you read on, you will see how toxins also affect the autonomic nervous system.

Positive Thinking I now live my life turning negatives into positives. In retrospect, I was blessed with a positive outlook and a supportive forward-thinking physician like Dr. Kailin. However, to demonstrate how positive thinking changed my life, my story must first illustrate how negatives first manifested themselves.

Have You Had These Thoughts Too? I laughed at Rachel Carson's warning about pesticides.[1] I scorned people who were always sick with allergies. To me, allergies and hypochondria were synonymous. I scoffed at health warnings against smoking, soft drinks and junk foods. I used all the clichés you probably do: "This does not apply to me; I am a healthy athlete. Besides, if I have to live that cautiously, avoiding everything I love to eat and do, forget it. Life isn't worth living under those circumstances."

CHANGING PERSPECTIVES

Then It Happened Nearly simultaneously, I sustained an automobile accident, a kitchen stove gas leak, a leaking oil burner and direct exposure to insecticides. Prior to these, I felt so physically strong and robust that it took all four exposures to reduce me to life-threatening illness.

I was fortunate. By accident I discovered Dr. Kailin, who helped me find the long road back and start my career as an author. Many doctors encouraged me to tell how I changed my lifestyle, progressing from healthy athletic activity to life-threatening illness and returning to health, happiness and productivity. I was told my recovery offers hope to the most sensitive patient. My story may also be an eye-opener to you healthy people who believe this illness could not possibly happen to you.

Need for Prevention My illness illustrates the need for using preventive measures and why even minor symptoms should not be ignored. In 1958, I was asymptomatic, but after my annual physical, my physician told me his examination of my nose suggested a possibility of a slight allergy, so minor I did not need an allergist.

Two years later, I experienced a mild reaction to deodorant and a few other things, but I ignored the symptoms because my doctor told me I would be labeled a hypochondriac.

In a few months, physicians who tried to help me were puzzled by symptoms I could no longer ignore. An ophthalmologist suggested that eyestrain caused my blurred vision. My general practitioner said my chronic fatigue was caused by overwork. An internist-allergist said my problem could be spastic colon.

Ironically, when I finally went to another allergist I was given dust shots that contained preservatives. While I am still allergic to dust, some of my worst offenders are preservatives, especially phenol, which was in the dust extract. The test was worthless since I reacted to the preservative.

In retrospect I recognize that the symptoms were worse and lasted longer when I was under pressure from my job, but they followed the same pattern week after week. As this book proceeds you will repeatedly observe that enhancing your

9

Accordion Reserve© is equivalent to reducing both emotional and toxic stress.

By 1966, I was so ill that I was unable to tolerate a normal diet. I had to relocate my living quarters eight times in three years in search of an environment I could tolerate. Over an eight-year period, my condition had progressed from a simple reaction to a semi-invalid state of complex allergies and severe chemical sensitivities.

Hindsight I never fully understood the mechanism that caused my collapse until Alan and I experienced the richness of the Accordion Reserve© model. There can be no question that my sensitivity advanced from mild to severe because I had so depleted my reserve. Following the concepts of the Ecologic-Oriented History, we will examine my habits at that time to discover what happened.

Foods I indulged my insatiable hunger for beef, potatoes, bread and sweets, especially milk chocolate. When my sensitivity was diagnosed, of course I tested most positive for beef, potatoes, wheat, sugar and chocolate (see Chapter 17).

Chemicals I always wrapped everything in plastic — my foods, the contents of my closets and drawers: shoes, gloves, hats, sweaters and coats. I introduced other chemicals into my bedroom by installing shelves for books, magazines, copy paper, carbon paper, felt-tip markers and other toxic office supplies. Later I learned that ink, plastics and pesticides induced my most severe chemical reactions.

HAD I KNOWN THE Accordion Reserve©

Before I was properly diagnosed and because I am a delayed reactor, I was unable to recognize what was really bothering me – what was causing symptoms. For example, I wondered what made me ill when I was conducting business banquets and dinner meetings. Because I was always seated at the dais surrounded by floral arrangements, I assumed I was allergic to flowers. Later I discovered that it was not the <u>flowers</u> but the <u>insecticide</u> <u>on</u> the flowers that caused my problems. Unfortunately, years later after my immune system was so challenged, I developed "classic" allergies (plants, trees, grass, etc.).

A LESSON TO BE LEARNED

Reflecting on my misfortunes, I can now laugh at the following events that caused so many problems. With bittersweet emotion, I laugh with the proverbial "lump in my throat and a tear in my eye" because, at the time, these incidents were very distressing. I was already teetering on the brink and didn't know it. Hopefully, even if you seem to be symptom-free, you can avoid my pitfalls by using a measure of caution.

I used to say: "I never had any allergies except for a slight sensitivity to some deodorants." In 1966, when I was furnishing a new apartment, my sister suggested that, since I had a mild sensitivity, I should buy an acrylic carpet instead of my chosen woolen one. "Besides," she said, "it will cost you less money." Being a practical person, I decided on acrylic. Nine months later, I was diagnosed severely sensitive to acrylic and other synthetics, but not to wool.

For my draperies, I chose beautiful antique silk shantung. The interior decorator suggested I could save money by lining the drapes with special material to protect them from sun damage. I later learned that silk was no problem, but I was highly sensitive to the chemically-treated lining.

My custom-designed sleep sofa was treated to resist stains "to save the cost" of frequent cleaning. The stain-resistant mixture made the fabric so toxic that ten years later I still could not sit on the sofa, which had been moved to a relative's home.

In a previous book, my Simon & Schuster editor prevented me from using the product name "Scotch Guard™" because of the liability risk. More recently, it was reported in *Business Week* that the manufacturer became aware that "tiny amounts of a chemical 3M had made for 40 years were showing up in blood drawn from people living all across the country, even in places far from 3M factories."[2] When the information became public, it was announced that the product was being re-formulated. How many thousands of readers could I have helped if I had used the name "Scotch Guard[TM]" in the 1979 edition of *Coping with Your Allergies.*[3]

BECOMING A DETECTIVE

Looking for Patterns In retrospect, my new apartment was not the only factor that caused my immune system to collapse. My decline began years earlier when, as a student in New York City, I was living in a building located in a deteriorating area. The locals were careless about cleanliness. I persuaded the exterminator to spray my apartment whenever he serviced my building. I did not want bugs from other apartments migrating into my apartment.

While the spraying was effective in reducing the bug population, the surviving bugs became resistant. Unfortunately, over time, it had the opposite effect on me. I learned the hard way. I hope you will heed the warning from my experience and, at least in your own home, control insects with less-toxic procedures. (See Integrated Pest Management in the Glossary.)

Pattern Search Uncovers Forgotten Clues The following incident concerns the need to protect yourself from polluted environments. My first teaching job was in a private boarding school situated in a beautiful wooded area. The school became overrun with insects and small animals. Over a long weekend the school building was sealed so that it could be fumigated. The exterminator called it "bombing."

Years later, after Dr. Randolph treated me, I realized that those toxins affected many students and faculty. I vividly remember many discipline problems subsequent to the pesticide treatment. One example was a twelve-year-old boy who threw a chair across the room. The piano teacher broke out with such a painful rash on her hands that she had to wear gloves so that she could play the piano. At the time I was a well-conditioned athlete, and I did not experience any immediate reactions. I thought I was healthy, but was I?

A short time after the "bombing," fatigue set in. My sleep pattern changed. I awakened in a death-like state. I couldn't wake up on time, and I required afternoon naps. I had unexplained muscle pains, which I ignored. I attributed soreness and fatigue to excessive strenuous exercise, yet I continued to push myself in many athletic endeavors with the students, after I completed my teaching responsibilities.

In retrospect, my body was telling me something. My athletic pursuits were a way to rid myself of toxins. I did not know then that the toxins were causing early symptoms associated with Autonomic Neuropathy and Chronic Fatigue Syndrome.

Alan keeps emphasizing: "Are you healthy or just symptom free?" Instead of being as self-certain as I was, don't discover after-the-fact that you too had an early warning and ignored it.

And "now you know the Rest of the Story."[4]

THE SPREADING PHENOMENON[5]

Paralysis was not the only manifestation of the toxic damage to my central nervous system. I had all the symptoms of what is now well known as toxic encephalopathy (brain damage caused by toxins). My immune system and autonomic nervous system were also adversely affected.

Within five minutes of exposure to a printed page, my vision was impaired. Plastic electrical equipment (phone, radio, television and electric blanket) offgased fumes, which distorted my vision and hearing and triggered right-sided muscle pain. My digestive system rejected all foods I previously tolerated and many I had never eaten before. For two years I survived on twenty exotic foods — wild game such as buffalo, quail and hippopotamus.

During those periods when I was confined to bed, I was unable to watch television or listen to a radio. I began to write my first book in pencil, since ink also distorted my vision. Even though I had severe pains in my right side and paralysis on my left side, I was fortunate to use part of my brain and my right hand. I decided that with the right mental attitude I could always be productive. But I must say how grateful I am that I found Dr. Randolph and Dr. Kailin before pesticides and other toxic chemicals permanently destroyed me.

The Accordion Reserve©
IS MY PAST, PRESENT AND FUTURE

Years ago I was told I would have to live in isolation. "Move away from suburbia," some said — away from society and its pollution. In my case they were wrong. However, for some highly sensitive reactors who suffer from toxic overexposure a move may be necessary for a period of recuperation and building up one's energy reserves. Dr. Randolph always emphasized the need for a daily eight-hour period in a pure environment.

My search is documented in snippets inserted throughout this book. My efforts were a struggle. I learned through trial and error which stringent methods would help and which would harm me. I tried them all, at least the ones I could afford. Some procedures I invented, some I stumbled on, some I learned from other patients and from medical courses I attended.

To rejuvenate and replenish my body tolerance I still live in the specially outfitted home that helped me recover from advanced ETI. My home is my "oasis"[6] that helps me function in the pollution-filled world of suburbia. Thanks to Serendipity and my chance meeting with Alan, we found the missing link, The *Accordion Reserve*[©], which has speeded my recovery and can do the same for those already sensitive as well as prevent ETI in the rest of you.

Do I still have setbacks when my nervous or immune systems are again challenged? Yes. But with most episodes my time for recovery is brief, and my tolerance to challenges is fortunately much higher.

Do I still have to be concerned about indoor air quality? Doesn't everyone? Do I live in a Bubble? No, and I can prove it. You be the Judge. Because I refused to become a vegetable protected in a Bubble, I searched for my personal "cure."

IN PARTS III - VII YOU WILL FIND STEPS TO HELP YOU ACHIEVE SIMILAR RESULTS.

I wrote before that "You should live in a Bubble" is incorrect advice. As a result of my search for a cure, I pursued three new careers:

* *Teacher (stress reduction and visualization)*
  Parts III and IV describe Visualization and Meditative/Relaxation Healing, which I now teach to patients and non-patients alike, and recommend methods I used to improve my health and environment (Parts V-VII).
* *Author* This is my seventh book, all reporting the results of my research and experiences.

* <u>*Environmental Medicine Counselor*</u> To maintain current knowledge in Environmental Medicine and other modalities, I accumulated over 2000 hours of Continuing Medical Education credits. My travels have taken me to seminars in USA, Canada, Great Britain and Germany, as well as lecturing and teaching doctors and their staff, and patients. In addition, I have traveled to the Caribbean, Mexico, Nova Scotia, Ireland and Scotland, sleeping in conditions as diverse as thatched huts, beds & breakfasts and five-star hotels.

CAUTION! Today there are many books on ETI, but for years, my books were the major source in patient education. At first I was flattered when readers told me that my book was their "bible." However, something happened to show me how dangerous that thought was, and how I had to correct it.

I was lecturing to Dr. William Rea's patients in his Environmentally Controlled Unit (ECU).[7] He walked in and laughingly commented, "Has Natalie told you about her chocolate binges?" The class seemed amused, as I shared funny incidents, which defined my struggle with chocolate addiction.

At the end, a newly arrived patient approached and said, "I'm so glad I met you. I have been reading your book *Coping with Your Allergies,* and I thought you were some kind of a nut. I'm relieved to find that you're a normal human being. I thought I would never again live in the 'Real World.'"

THUNDER AND LIGHTNING! Something was wrong! Although I have written, "Don't try to be a one hundred percenter," readers were missing the point. That message needs more repetition, more clarification. <u>You don't have to live in a bubble!</u> You have to "play the Accordion" to increase your energy reserve and create an oasis.[8] I did, and I am blessed once again.

♪♪♪♪♪

[1] Carson R. 1962. *Silent Spring.* 40th Edition, Houghton Mifflin, Boston.

[2] Weber J. "3M's big cleanup: Why it decided to pull the plug on its best-selling stain repellant." *Business Week*, June 5, 2000, p. 96-98.

[3] Golos N, Golbitz FG. 1979, 1986. *Coping with Your Allergies.* Simon and Schuster, New York.

[4] Harvey Paul. Radio journalist. *"The Rest of the Story."*

[5] Rea WJ. 1992. *Chemical Sensitivity,* Volume 1. Lewis Press, Boca Raton.

[6] Rea WJ. 1992-1997. *Chemical Sensitivity.*

[7] Rea WJ. 1997. *Chemical Sensitivity,* Volume 4.

[8] See New Hope, Appendix D.

3

ALAN'S STORY -
Thwarted:
An Illness Waiting to Happen

♫♫♫♫♫

I always thought I was healthy. However, since 1996 my concepts about health and my practice of medicine have been changed by the teachings of a doctor I never met, Dr. Theron Randolph.

As you read in the Foreword one of Dr. Randolph's major contributions to the field of medicine was his patient questionnaire now called the "Ecologic-Oriented History." It emphasizes the influence of environmental exposure and the possible link between exposure and the onset of health complaints.

The effective results of Dr. Randolph's methods are illustrated by my discovery of major causes of illness onset for three of my patients. During the history taking of one patient I recognized that her complaints were similar to two other patients, all three of whom were teachers in the same school. On further investigation, I discovered that at distinct times in different years each of the three taught in the same classroom. This observation led to a series of studies that identified the cause of illness resulting from the adverse classroom environment.

WARNING SIGNALS

Soon I questioned my own patterns of decline. Since my early twenties, I have been an avid runner, beginning with a few miles a day in the early years, and gradually increasing to marathon running in my early forties. However, my health gradually declined for twenty-five years despite excellent cardiovascular conditioning.

In my early twenties, I suffered a knee injury from running and chronic rashes from sun exposure. Later, I developed regular upper respiratory infections

19

(nearly every 3 months), including a bout with pneumonia.

In my early forties, I developed exercise-induced asthma, which required increasing doses of medication, but I continued running very successfully. Soon after running my first marathon, I suffered my first major injury, which affected my left knee and hamstring. This was followed by a series of back, hip, calf and ankle injuries.

During my second marathon, I suffered fluid and weight loss, dehydration, lack of energy and extreme dizziness in spite of sufficient conditioning, training and fluid intake. Thereafter I continued my decline, experiencing periodic injuries (including a stress fracture), runner's diarrhea, increased blood pressure, mood changes, chronic stuffy nose and sleep apnea. These conditions required medications. Frustrated by my worsening health and the inability of medications to halt this decline, I began to study vitamins and found some success in relieving these conditions. But it was not until I began connecting to the environmental medicine community that I finally discovered the path to full recovery.

The Biggest Journey of My Life

In Chapter 1, Natalie told you how we met at Shady Grove Adventist Hospital Grand Rounds, presented by Dr. William Rea. His talk was one of the most memorable I have ever heard. He was reviewing the ground regulating system (GRS) and its impact on information transfer throughout the body. Dr. Rea's presentation was my first connection linking anatomy to acupuncture and the body's bioelectrical system.

After the meeting, Natalie invited me to other gatherings of environmentally oriented health care practitioners. Natalie didn't realize it at the time, but I was a "doubting Thomas." But I finally crumbled under her persistence and attended Dr. Rea's meeting in February 1996 – "The 14th Annual International Symposium on Man and His Environment."

I was so skeptical that I continued to say to my wife Ruth: "I'm going, but I won't believe a word of it!" Much to my surprise, I found myself asking many questions about case presentations. They reminded me of some of my patients who never seemed to recover. I had been "spinning my wheels" trying to help them.

20

Powerless, I was motivated to discover a new approach (for me) to assess and treat such resistant health problems. My biggest journey was beginning.

My Personal Body Awareness In Part IV, Chapters 10, 11 and 12 Natalie discusses some methods she taught me about Body Awareness, breathing and visualization. She showed me how she teaches patients to ground themselves and connect with their energy. Techniques of breathing and meditation unlocked a part of me that I never knew existed.

As we worked together I validated my intuitive 6th sense. Through the years, for example, when I suddenly thought of someone's name, that person would invariably contact me within days. I have finally discovered significant reasons for these occurrences, which I can now usually control with my energy.

As Natalie led me through a meditation exercise, she explained how patients use her voice to maintain focus on the meditation while letting their minds wander into their own symbols and deeper meditative state. So, I allowed my mind to take flight. I listened to Natalie's voice and was aware of it throughout. As my mind wandered, I suddenly sensed the image of an accordion. It was so vivid that I shared this image with her.

Fascinated by this extraordinary encounter, my mind flourished with a new image nearly every time I meditated, especially when I was running. But I always returned to the image of the accordion, which remained as powerful as on its first occurrence. Our discussions would always return to the image of the accordion and its impact on our concerns about environmental health. During other meditative sequences I was able again to experience the beauty and power of the accordion until it finally evolved into our working model, the Accordion Reserve©.

A Powerful Message The accordion was striking in a way I could not yet comprehend. Six months later I related the accordion experiences to my Aunt Ruth. A 90-year-old concert pianist, she still performs publicly. "Did you know that your grandfather loved to play the accordion?" I was amazed. "No," I replied. She continued, "He stopped playing a year before he died, and I never understood why he stopped playing it, because he always had such energy when he played."

21

I never met my grandpa Abe, who died three years before I was born. Out of respect, my parents named me for him.

I surmise that this message has two possible explanations: energy was transported across time with no real time boundaries or through the genetic pool information was transported to me through my father.

Natalie believes that meditative images and symbols are messages from our Guiding Force. Whatever the mechanism or symbolism, I was blessed to become aware of this powerful image.

Fusion The pieces of the puzzle came together after the most significant workshop and conference that I have ever attended: Dr. William Rea's "The 15th Annual International Symposium on Man and His Environment" in 1997. The unifying topic was bioelectricity. There were many presentations: concepts of images, dispersal of energy and recognizing variability in the autonomic nervous system.

Like my experience at the previous symposium, I was impressed with the wealth of scientific information presented. I was so excited that I called Natalie at the end of the day's events. In a later chapter, Natalie reveals why she missed the meeting but sensed that I was going to call her. After that call we began to meet in earnest.

My Personal Ecologic-Oriented History (EOH)

In retrospect, knowing and understanding how I pursued my recovery from illnesses and injuries described in Warning Signals, it occurred to me that I have made significant progress in understanding nutrition, illness in general, but specifically my own personal health.

In the last 3 years I have been to hell and back, professionally, personally and socially. I believe that these adversities would have overwhelmed me had I not learned what we present in our book.

What follows is an example of my EOH. For my patients I recommend that they create a chronological time-line of important exposures (e.g. renovations at work or at home) and correlate them with their own symptoms. For simplicity of reading this material, I wrote my EOH in paragraph rather than in chart format.

During childhood I was exposed to mercury from a coal-burning furnace, pesticides from gardening, mothballs, cigarette smoke, as well as formaldehyde and solvents from chemistry and biology labs (which continued into college and medical school). During college I suffered a neck injury, which was never treated.

Later exposures included solvents from furniture refinishing, pesticides from gardening, volatile organic chemicals from wallpapering and painting, solvents and sawdust from household construction projects, gasoline fumes from yard-work and diesel fumes from my cars.

Even my homes have been toxic, exposing me to residual pesticides from the garden, diesel fumes from the car and attached garages, mold from basement flooding, chemical soup from basement refinishing, new carpet fumes, varnish from hardwood floor refinishing, smoke from improperly vented wood-burning fireplaces and mold from roof leaks. Given these toxic exposures over a lifetime, my knowledge of environmental medicine has finally allowed me to clearly understand why my health was in decline.

MY TRANSFORMATION

I am amazed at how I've changed over these last seven years. I experienced so many extraordinary events, revelations and images. Their impact allowed me to endure some of the most trying negative events in my life. Those adversities remind me that my insights into how I now practice medicine were conceived in discovering how I "thwarted the illness waiting to happen."

♫♫♫♫♫

PART II

Fountains
of
Ideas and Creativity

NEW APPROACHES
to HEALTH

4

EXTENDING THE PHILOSOPHY
OF ENVIRONMENTAL HEALTH

Prologue

You can better understand today's concept of a healthy body if you learn about Environmental Medicine (EM), the branch of medicine that examines everything you breathe, eat, drink, touch, smell, sense and feel. You are your environment, and you exist within your environment.

FOUR PERSPECTIVES OF ENVIRONMENTAL MEDICINE

Fundamental to learning about Environmentally Triggered Illness (ETI) and Environmental Health (EH) are the teachings of the late Dr. Theron Randolph, the pioneer of EM. He introduced his concepts in *Human Ecology and Susceptibility to the Chemical Environment.*[1] His ideas of understanding acute and chronic exposures were expanded by Dr. William Rea. Dr. Doris Rapp has raised public conscience about EM with her books and appearances on popular TV shows. From her own encounters with ETI, author Natalie Golos has documented personal insights and experiences and is a living example of how to overcome ETI through avoidance and stress management.

Dr. Theron Randolph In the foreword of *Coping with Your Allergies*[2] Dr. Randolph wrote that educating patients with ETI requires a tremendous amount of time. Most often, people do not understand how they get so ill.

Dr. Randolph explained that the likelihood of developing ETI depends on an individual's acute and chronic environmental exposures, major infections, hormonal shifts, sleep deprivation and

27

the genetic tendency to develop allergies. While acute exposures are easy to identify, Dr. Randolph addressed chronic low-grade exposures as a cause of illness for housewives exposed to gas-burning stoves and for many workers exposed to other volatile hydrocarbons (examples include paints, sprays, insecticides, gasoline and perfumes). *Energy – the Essence of Environmental Health* is a tribute to Dr. Randolph and the way he taught doctors and patients.

A major influence on Dr. Randolph was the research of Dr. Hans Selye regarding stress and its effects on human systems. According to Selye,[3] stress — emotional, allergic or toxic — will generate specific responses in the body.

Thinking of negative situations can trigger the same response as locking the diaphragm or holding one's breath. When the body is stressed, it becomes more sensitive and reactive to allergens. Allergic people know that as stress increases, their allergic symptoms increase.

Dr. Randolph focused on reducing environmental toxins in homes and work places of allergy sufferers. Other researchers emphasized the need to reduce the threshold for emotional stress. Others recognized the need to learn to discipline one's breathing and imagination to avoid creating self-inflicted tension.

Dr. William J. Rea   In his four-volume set *Chemical Sensitivity*,[4] Dr. Rea explained environmental exposures in terms of a body being like a rain barrel that fills with toxins. Before the barrel overflows, you may be developing ETI and not know it. When the barrel finally overflows, symptoms begin, first in one organ or organ system, then another. Unless the barrel is drained, illness develops in a unique pattern for each individual, even if exposures are relatively similar. *Chemical Sensitivity* is accepted worldwide as a primary text for EM Practitioners.

Dr. Doris Rapp   In *Is This Your Child's World?*,[5] Dr. Rapp directed the public's attention to poor indoor air quality in schools where children and their teachers spend their days. She used the term

"Allergy Tension Fatigue Syndrome" to describe children who react their school environment.

Dr. Rapp suggested that Attention Deficit Hyperactivity Disorder is possibly an over-diagnosed condition because exposure factors were not considered during diagnostic evaluation. She suggested that many children might not need Ritalin® because after evaluation they could improve with avoidance of exposures, modified nutrition and allergy treatments called provocation/neutralization.

Dr. Rapp has authored many other books including the *New York Times* best seller, *Is This Your Child?*[6]

♫♫♫♫♫

Natalie Golos Through Natalie's writings, most notably the internationally acclaimed *Coping with Your Allergies*, she offered herself as an example of how to overcome ETI. Over the years I have witnessed Natalie's efforts to recruit leading EM Physicians to help her teach local doctors and other health professionals – members of the Mid-Atlantic Environmental Medicine Network, which she founded. She remains committed to spreading the word about ETI and EH and is the inspiration for the current volume.
♫♫♫♫♫

---

[1] Randolph TG. 1962. *Human Ecology and Susceptibility to the Chemical Environment.* Charles C Thomas, Publisher, Springfield, IL.

[2] Golos N, Golbitz FG. 1979. *Coping with Your Allergies.* Simon & Schuster, New York. 1986. Fireside Edition.

[3] Selye H. 1976. Forty years of stress research: principal remaining problems and misconceptions. *Canadian Med Assn Jl* 115:53-6.

[4] Rea, WJ. *Chemical Sensitivity.* 1992-1997. Volumes 1-4. Lewis Press, Boca Raton, FL.

[5] Rapp, D. 1996. *Is This Your Child's World?* Bantam Books, New York.

[6] Rapp, D. 1991. *Is This Your Child?* Morrow, New York.

5

THE ACCORDION RESERVE© -
Our Working Model

Prologue

With apologies to Shakespeare's "If music be the food of love," we also equate music to the "Food of Healing." Begin thinking of your body as a musical instrument and you as the composer/conductor/choreographer preparing a symphony of optimum Environmental Health (EH). Our musical analogy unfolds as each chapter builds until you become a master of your health. Building on concepts briefly outlined in Chapter 4, we present for the first time in writing an extended idea that unifies Mind/body/soul/spirit with fundamentals of Environmental Medicine (EM). Our symbol is the Accordion Reserve©.

By the time you complete this book you will appreciate how:

*   The Accordion Reserve© represents your ever-changing energy level
*   The Accordion Reserve© represents the strength of your body's tolerance to the environment
*   The Accordion Reserve© influences every phase of your health
*   Our working model is a practical instructional tool, using visualization to help you feel and use your healing energy.

THE ACCORDION - A DYNAMIC MUSICAL INSTRUMENT

Shapiro describes the accordion as "The Joygiver". "No other reed instrument on the face of the earth is as versatile as the accor-

dion.   It can play melody, harmony and rhythm simultaneously."[1]
We call it the Accordion Reserve© (**Figure 5-1**).

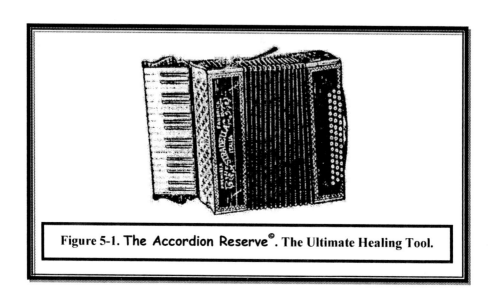

Figure 5-1. The Accordion Reserve©. The Ultimate Healing Tool.

VIBRATION - THE UNIVERSAL FORCE

Mothers Know Best Do you remember when your mother
told you: "Put on your jacket. You'll get cold and catch pneumonia!"? She was intuitively correct, even before we scientifically knew
that the immune system is influenced by the weather. In a similar
way, we intuitively know that we react to the energetic forces of nature such as wind, radiation, electromagnetic fields, chemicals and
those generated by living organisms.

Vibrational Energy According to scholars, energy is generated from movement of vibrating particles. In the absence of particles, which is a vacuum, there is no vibration. The expression "you
don't live in a vacuum" is both figurative and literal. Since you cannot
exist in a vacuum, you are constantly exposed to vibrational energy.

VIBRATION PRODUCES MUSIC

Musical Lessons from Nature Listen to nature and learn to hear the whistle of the wind, the crunch of an apple and the ripple of waves breaking against the shore. You have experienced vibrational energy. Listen to the sounds of your body and tune into your own unique vibrational energy. Feel your body's vibrations as you follow our musical theme.

THE ACCORDION - MIND/BODY/SOUL/SPIRIT ANALOGY

Our working model illustrates that both your body's vibrational energy and environmental factors must be considered to understand Environmentally Triggered Illness (ETI) and to maintain or restore Environmental Health (EH). The accordion represents ever-changing vibration and movement. Human energy parallels these changes – mental, physical, intuitive and spiritual – in other words Mind/body/soul/spirit.

THE ACCORDION RESERVE© - OUR WORKING MODEL

Environmental Health A relatively contaminant-free environment (avoiding or eliminating molds, dust, toxic factors, etc.) + peak energy (good habits — sleep, exercise, diet, deep-breathing techniques and other stress-reduction factors) = expanded Accordion Reserve©. This is increased Body Tolerance. (**Figure 5-2**).

Environmentally Triggered Illness Accumulated toxic environmental factors + diminished energy factors = collapsing Accordion Reserve©. This represents reduced Body Tolerance. (**Figure 5-3**). This illustrates complex illnesses such as Chronic Fatigue Syndrome, Gulf War Syndrome, Fibromyalgia, Chemical Sensitivities, Vasculitis, Autonomic Neuropathy and other forms of ETI.

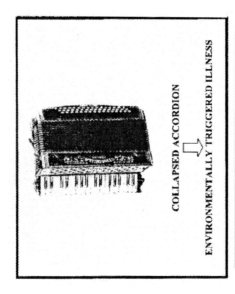

COLLAPSED ACCORDION

ENVIRONMENTALLY TRIGGERED ILLNESS

Figure 5-3. Environmentally Triggered Illness — Accumulated toxic environmental factors + diminished energy factors = collapsed *Accordion Reserve*, representing reduced Body Tolerance. This illustrates complex illnesses such as Chronic Fatigue Syndrome, Gulf War Syndrome, Fibromyalgia, Chemical Sensitivities, Vasculitis, Autonomic Neuropathy and other forms of ETL.

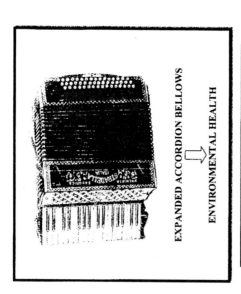

EXPANDED ACCORDION BELLOWS

ENVIRONMENTAL HEALTH

Figure 5-2. Environmental Health — A relatively contaminant-free environment (avoiding or eliminating molds, dust, toxic factors, etc.) + peak energy (good habits — sleep, exercise, diet, deep-breathing techniques and other stress-reduction factors). This represents increased Body Tolerance.

DETAILS

The researcher, professional and the curious can turn to Part VIII: Professional Challenges at the conclusion of the main text to explore the breadth of studies that are possible in further assessment of the autonomic nervous system and the Accordion. To facilitate the flow of the text, we provide an overview in the paragraphs that follow.

ENVIRONMENTAL FACTORS

From Your Environment to You Think of your body as a factory functioning in an outside environment, continuously interacting with external factors whenever you breathe, eat, touch or use our senses. Your body processes exposures in various ways: modifying and then eliminating them by breathing, urinating, defecating, sweating, tearing, menstruating, lactating or bleeding. Toxins may also be stored. Both toxins and physical factors (radiation, sun exposure, etc.) may result in temporary or permanent changes to structures or functions in your body.

Internal Body Communications Internal body influences are represented by complex interactions among cells and its substructures, genetic code, organs and organ systems. Your body communicates along pathways such as nerves and blood vessels, and uses many types of messengers like hormones, neurotransmitters and chemical mediators. In a newly released article zoologist Matt Ridley[2] hypothesized that the important complex interaction between external/internal environmental factors and personal experiences influences how your genes function and *vice versa*.

ENERGY FACTORS

Your Vibrations at Work Energy is derived from a combination of external and internal factors, which are generated from the dynamic interactions of Sleep, Exercise, Nutrition and Relationships. Relationships include those with yourself, with others, with your in-

35

ternal and external environments and with your Guiding Force. In addition, your Belief System influences your Energy in a positive way.

> _You Are a Part of Your Environment_ You are in a complex relationship with your environment, and therefore you are a part of it. Hence, there is constant, dynamic and total environmental influence throughout your life, and each individual's cumulative interactions are unique. While symptom patterns tend to repeat themselves, each individual takes a different path to arrive at that state at any moment in time.

Mind/body/soul/spirit

Recalling the **Accordion - Mind/body/soul/spirit** Analogy, you can appreciate that **Mind/body/soul/spirit** spans the entire Accordion.

Natalie's discussion which follows in Parts III and IV will explore the many rhythms, refrains and variations that apply to **Mind/body/soul/spirit**. Part III teaches breathing, **Body Awareness** and conditioning in Chapters 7-9. Part IV introduces the new technique "**Playing with Your Aura©**" (a **Mind/body/soul/spirit**-expanding experience).

As you read Part III and Part IV, Natalie demonstrates that you have frequencies in your body that led us to the musical analogy – Your **Accordion Reserve©** = Your Vibrational Energy Reserve.

HEALTHY OR SYMPTOM-FREE?

Your Vibrational Energy Reserve is a major factor in your EH. Because the **Accordion Reserve©** represents the unknown quantity of your constantly changing ability to tolerate stresses of many diverse body functions, your **Accordion Reserve©** may be smaller than you realize. Your reserve may be gradually shrinking without noticeable signs. What are the consequences? Are you "Healthy" or "Symptom-free"? These words do not express the same concept. You may not be truly healthy, even if you have no symptoms.

When **does** your Accordion's Bellows collapse enough to allow for occasional symptoms? Unfortunately, nobody knows how to give a quantitative answer. In any event, this book will provide you with information so you can develop **Body Awareness skills** that will allow you to recognize declining health before or at the earliest onset of symptoms (**see Parts III and IV**). In other words, you can learn how to recognize a collapsing **Accordion Reserve©**.

At the other end of the spectrum are **people with severe manifestations of ETI**. Unfortunately for you, your **Accordion Reserve©** is severely collapsed and symptoms occur with minor provocation. **Body Awareness is even more important for you!** Preventing further deterioration is crucial by initiating protection and repair skills that you will learn as you join us in this musical journey.

SUMMARY

Energy and vibration co-exist. The presence of Energy implies that vibrations are also present. The presence of vibrations promotes music.

Your body contains vibrations and is therefore a musical instrument. This premise is the basis for our musical analogy.

Our working model the **Accordion Reserve©** predicts multiple **Energy** and **Environmental** variables (**the Handles**) with dynamic interactions. The result is an ever-changing set of symptoms with changing dimensions (**the Bellows**).

Symptoms occur in patterns recognized as diseases, conditions, disorders or syndromes. Illness patterns may be less discrete than previously recognized by conventional mainstream medicine.

The following conclusions derive from the above tenets:

1) The Accordion Reserve© organizes data collected from an Ecologic-Oriented History, forming the basis for accurate diagnosis and treatment.

2) A markedly collapsed Bellows represents severe ETI, and a collapsing Bellows suggests evolving ETI.

3) Continuing expansion of the Bellows represents improving EH.

4) Treatments for symptoms are predicted as a result of identifying underlying etiologies when evaluating the Environment and Energy Handles.

5) The Accordion Reserve© represents Mind/body/soul/spirit and reflects the influence of vibrations on your existence.

6) External Environmental and Energy Factors can result in positive and negative impact on the size and movement of the Accordion.

7) Internal Energy and Environmental Factors result in positive and negative impact on the size and movement of the Accordion.
   a) Stored Internal Factors, representing negative Energy or Vibrations, cause the Accordion to collapse. These factors may be toxins, remembered negative thoughts or traumas. When released, they may trigger symptoms until eliminated.
   b) These stored Internal Factors may contribute to symptoms when External Factors appear to be adequately controlled.
   c) These stored Internal Factors must be reconnoitered when a diagnosis remains elusive.

---

[1] Shapiro M. 1995. *Planet Squeezebox*, p. 5.
[2] Ridley, M. "What Makes You Who You Are," *Time Magazine*, June 2, 2003, p. 54-63.

6

THE AUTONOMIC NERVOUS SYSTEM -
Validating the Accordion Reserve ©

Prologue

Articles, books and chapters have been written about the autonomic nervous system (ANS). As individuals, we intuitively know that the ANS exists, yet do we really know how it relates to our overall health?

We all know about Stress, and we've heard the expression "Flight or Fight." This concept is fundamental to understanding the ANS, yet applying it to our own health is hard to do. It is hard for health care providers to assess when you are under stress and even harder to assess why you are under stress!

In this chapter, we lay the foundation for how the **Accordion Reserve**© relates to the ANS. In Part VIII: Professional Challenges, we provide more detailed information for the researcher, professional and the curious among you.

THE AUTONOMIC NERVOUS SYSTEM

"The autonomic nervous system is involved in virtually all disease."[1] As you will soon discover, the **Accordion Reserve**© reflects the function of the ANS.

<u>*Sympathetic Nervous System (SNS)*</u> "Fright, then Flight or Fight" (3-F's) is the expression that describes how an organism survives. The phrase implies instantaneous problem solving without thinking about it. In other words, the SNS responds to stress.

You discover an immediate threat. In order to protect yourself, you must **expend energy** to restore yourself. Your blood pressure goes up, heart rate quickens, blood sugar rises, muscles contract vigorously, you develop gooseflesh as your skin turns cold or you pee in your pants. This is the SNS at work.

Parasympathetic Nervous System (PSNS) Energy conservation, healing and a return to normal are duties of the PSNS. You cannot survive for long if you continue to expend energy at intensive rates. So your PSNS turns down your heart rate, helps you go to sleep, gets you to breathe gently and helps your organs function.

Communication in the ANS Nerves are specially structured to release messengers called neurotransmitters. There are many complex interactions between one nerve and the next, and between nerves and other cells of various organs. Keeping your body in balance depends on a highly integrated relationship between the PSNS and SNS.

STRESS

Usually you know when you feel stress by sensing the SNS working. And you probably feel stress is relieved when the PSNS takes over.

But there are times when stress remains uncorrected. In a sustained state, stress is damaging because the SNS becomes stronger and PSNS weakens, and they don't respond effectively to each other. Eventually, the SNS weakens as well. These impairments set the stage for illness.

You can relate to these basic principles because you remember when your mother developed breast cancer or your dad had a heart attack, soon after their parents died. Or your sister developed pneumonia after losing her job, or your baby developed a head injury after being overtired for days on end.[i]

SUSTAINED STRESS

When stress remains uncorrected for a while, you "get used to it." Scientists call this "adaptation."[2] Although you may feel okay, this condition is **not** normal. You may then develop a false sense of security because you have no apparent symptoms. Eventually small warnings creep in, then larger ones, until you need to get checked out. By this time your adaptive mechanisms are tired and failing. For most people, this stage means that your ANS is significantly unbalanced.

WARNING SIGNS

The best clues to ANS malfunction are when your energy is off. When you exercise do you feel exhilarated and refreshed? Do you exercise at all? Is your sleep comfortable and restful? Are your eating habits restorative and nutritious? Do you get along with yourself, your family, your peers and your superiors? Do you have and maintain a firm Belief System?

If you answer no to some of these questions, you might be surprised to discover that your ANS is unbalanced.

Early Recognition, Early Detection, Illness Prevention, Health Restored Wasn't it Ben Franklin who said: "An ounce of prevention is worth a pound of cure?" Only one problem – how do you detect that your ANS is in an early malfunctioning stage? Second, how do you discover why it is malfunctioning? And third, what do you do to correct it?

Enter Stage Left – the **Accordion Reserve**©.

---

[i] The complex interaction of the autonomic nervous system, hormonal system and immunologic system should be considered when dealing with stress. Many other resources are available to discuss these interactions.

The ANS — Accordion Reserve© Connection

♫♫♫♫♫

In Chapter 5, you learned the basics of the Accordion Reserve©. In my studies of Environmental Medicine, I learned that the ANS was a feature of complex illness. Yet I was never able to objectively measure its function. Then I learned about ANSAR®3 technology and began testing patients. The testing employed three different challenges or "Stress Tests." After observing the results for about 3 months, I observed the following:

* Challenge of the SNS correlated with a collapsing accordion.
* Challenge of the PSNS correlated with an expanding accordion.

It then logically followed that if the Accordion remained collapsed, a person would be under sustained stress. In other words, the SNS would be in overdrive and excess energy expenditure would continue. That is the setting in which illness is likely to occur.

The question is: How long can the Accordion continue to shrink before illness finally occurs? More importantly, how many times can you continue to adapt to stress without symptoms?

Did it occur to you that each attempt at adaptation was an effort by your PSNS to overcome your SNS?

♫♫♫♫♫

Checking In on Stress

You know what stress feels like in the short term. But what is causing the stress? You usually associate stress with "too much going on" as in "I've got too many deadlines," "My kids are acting up" and so on.

Did you remember to include stresses like it's too hot or cold or damp or cloudy (physical); smells like exhaust, cigarette smoke, perfumes, pesticide residues in your foods and air pollutants (chemicals); infections, mold and plants (biologic exposures)?

Did you remember to include travel across time zones, other sleep interferences, lack of or too much exercise, dieting or eating junk food?

Did you notice that the examples above are the list of items included on the environment and energy handles of the Accordion?

Stresses also include fever, dehydration, anemia and the presence of illness.

Did you also observe that treatments of illness might actually be stresses, even when symptoms of the treated condition seem to disappear? For example:

Treating
*   Strep throat with antibiotic changes the growth of good bacteria in your gastrointestinal tract.   Undesirable organisms then produce toxins which the liver cannot clear effectively.
*   Fever with acetominophen requires your liver to dispose of the fever-reducer. That function requires your body to use up glutathione, which depends on sufficient quantities of Vitamins B6 and B12, folic acid and the amino acid methionine.
*   Attention deficit disorder with a stimulant can cause appetite suppression, sleeplessness and slowed growth.[i]

In other words, when you discover "side effects" these are stress. And, as discussed above, sometimes the stress is hidden, like the first two examples.

---

[i] See Developmental Delay Resources (DDR), Appendix D.

CHECKING OUT HEALING

It follows from the above discussion that healing and maintaining health result from recognizing, reducing and resolving stress. When you make a trip to your health care provider, are you "putting your finger in the dike"? Are you relieving a symptom, while the long-term hidden stress is left unattended? Or are you substituting a hidden stress for the one that you just "cured"?

SYMPTOM RELIEF — SHORT-TERM GOAL; HEALING — LONG-TERM PLANNING

Everyone wants to feel well – NOW! As well you should! Please remember to ask yourself and your health care provider: Is this current illness part of a long-term problem — hidden asymptomatic stress? Discover if your ANS is in the early stages of decline and search for the reasons for that decline. Use the **Accordion Reserve**© model to provide a framework in your quest for Environmental Health.

---

[1] Low PA, Suarez GA, Benarroch EE. 1997. *Clinical Autonomic Disorders*: Classification and clinical evaluation. In *Clinical Autonomic Disorders,* 2nd Ed., Low PA (ed.) Lippincott-Raven Publishers, Philadelphia, PA.

[2] Selye H. 1946. The general adaptation syndrome and the diseases of adaptation. *J Allergy* 17:231.

[3] ANSAR Inc. 240 South Eighth St., Philadelphia, PA 19107, 1-888-883-7804, 215-922-6088.

PART III

Prerequisites to Energy Awareness

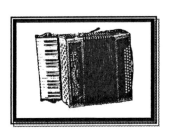

RELAXATION TECHNIQUES

7

BREATH OF HEALTH
- Phase I -
Balancing Your
Autonomic Nervous System

Prologue

♪♪♪♪♪

Saturday night, February 22, 1997. The phone rings. Saved by the bell! Saved from dark self-recriminating thoughts: I was brooding about missing the "15th Annual Symposium on Man and His Environment,"[1] seminars I have always attended. Why am I missing it this year of all years? Papers are presenting energy treatment modalities for the sensitive patient! That's the major focus of my "Meditation/Relaxation Healing!"

Why am I not in Texas with Alan? Why did I think of him? Oh! That must be Alan CALLING ME! The phone keeps ringing. As I answer, my mind shifts gears, bringing me back to the present. It **is** Alan, my co-author, very excited, calling to share his enthusiasm with me. Scientific papers included research studies that validate our method of using energy for healing, Alan's techniques for balancing energy with exercise and my "Meditation/Relaxation Healing."

♪♪♪♪♪

Please Note Although this and the next five chapters (Part III and Part IV) are separate, they can be considered as six phases, each phase building a foundation for the next. We have divided them because many readers will have varied experiences in one or more phases. We suggest you read them in order, reviewing phases familiar to you while concentrating on newer concepts. The progression may give you a better insight even to the phases familiar

47

to you. The unity will become apparent as we fashion the parts into a whole.

LISTENING - OUR DEFINITION

* "Listening" means "feeling, sensing, focusing or hearing with your ears." In other words, you are encouraged to take a sensory inventory of your body.

STRESS REDUCTION

Meditation/Relaxation Healing is the term we coin to describe our breathing techniques that balance the autonomic nervous system (ANS). **Meditation/Relaxation Healing** is the initial method for reducing stress because breathing has a major impact on improving the performance of the parasympathetic nervous system (PSNS).

Stress reduction is equivalent to expanding your Energy and improving the interaction between the sympathetic nervous system (SNS) and the PSNS. From previous chapters you learned that Energy enhancement is dependent upon improving sleep, exercise, nutrition and relationships.

♪♪♪♪

Exercise, breathing and relaxation techniques described here come from my personal experience and are suggested as an addition to and not a substitute for environmental control and proper diet. Additional procedures help reduce stress and enable you to lead a more normal and effective life without curtailing activities that are important to you.

♪♪♪♪

WHAT'S NEW ABOUT BREATHING?

Our technique of teaching breathing begins with a Meditation/Relaxation Healing program. There is nothing new about the need to train people to change breathing patterns. The latest trend however indicates the need to customize your breathing method in

48

accordance with the balance (or lack thereof) of your ANS. Your breathing technique must accommodate the difference in the strength of your SNS versus your PSNS. You learn by listening to your breathing.

Our method of teaching breathing has also been expanded to include visualization and the **Accordion Reserve**© from **PHASE I** on. As you proceed, you will learn how visualization helps break the habit of your mind controlling your breathing process.

Unhealthy Breathing Habits Most of us breathe properly at birth. However, a few infants experience "breath-holding spells." In toddler years, fearful children may get angry and stop breathing. As adults, media models emphasize having a "flat belly," which forcefully limits diaphragm motion.

When the mind attempts to control breathing it begins controlling functions of the ANS (heartbeat, circulation of blood, sweating and breathing).

DEVELOPING SENSITIVITY AWARENESS

Note to people who have received advanced training in Body Awareness — Yoga, Biofeedback, Chi Gong (Qi Gong), Meditation, T'ai-Chi, etc. — consider the next few pages as a review. You may generate ideas that will heighten your sensitivity and give you a greater grasp of the healing techniques that follow.

DEVELOPING PSNS BREATHING PATTERN

PSNS Breathing The soft area just below your sternum (the center of your rib cage) is where your diaphragm is attached to your abdomen. For simplicity, call this location "my diaphragm." Like a balloon filling with air, your belly (abdomen) inflates as it fills with air and deflates as it loses air. As you inhale with your hand on your belly, covering your navel, your diaphragm drops and expands, pushing your hand out. As you exhale, your diaphragm contracts, and your hand returns to its original position.

<u>*Comment*</u> All suggested procedures are in first person to help you develop your own program. By using the term "I feel," you are learning the first step to "listening" to your body.

PROCEDURE

* I stand straight, place my left hand on my belly and my right hand on my diaphragm.
* I feel my belly and diaphragm expanding and pushing out my hands as I slowly inhale through my nose to the count of 3.
* I feel my hand returning to starting position as I slowly breathe out through my mouth – to the count of 3. I rest to the count of 3.
* I repeat twice more to establish a pattern of 3 or sets of 3 – 6 – 9 – etc. Repetition in a pattern is the beginning of conditioning.

<u>*Comment*</u> The more you practice, the sooner your breathing pattern becomes habitual, increasing the effectiveness of your **Relaxation Breathing** (see below), the keystone to non-medical healing of the ANS and your overall state of health.

POSITIVELY OVERCOMING STRESS RESPONSES

As you develop awareness of your **PSNS Breathing**, you also become aware when stress causes you to lock your diaphragm. Instead of staying tense, you can return to natural breathing and **release your fear**, by putting one hand on your belly, the other on your diaphragm and focus on the movement of your hands. Breathe naturally. Do not force your breathing in this exercise.

When they are exposed to allergens many individuals lock their diaphragms, thereby increasing their sensitivity and reactions by activating their SNS, as described in PART VIII: Professional Challenges. Chronic activation of the SNS results in excessive stress hormone (e.g. cortisol) release, with the potential for deleterious health effects.

If you experience an offensive odor, most likely you automatically stop breathing, locking your diaphragm and setting off a "fright, then flight or fight" pattern. Learn to use PSNS Breathing to protect yourself and call it your Rapid Recovery.

Rapid Recovery Focusing on PSNS Breathing unlocks your diaphragm and releases your stress response. Stay relaxed and keep breathing (applying your hands to your abdomen, feeling the movement, as described above).

Visualize vapors leaving your body. You are then positively expanding your Energy Reserve, while slowing down what Alan calls "ANS Sympathetic Overdrive."

Apply similar visualizations to release any other fear-provoking trauma that you may encounter.

ENHANCING YOUR BREATHING TECHNIQUE

Whenever you have time to practice you can enhance your PSNS breathing by using the additional procedure below. Develop a pattern by repeating each step for a slow count of 3.

PROCEDURE

* Energize your nerve endings by lightly tapping your body with your fingertips, beginning with your arms (for a 3 count), then legs (for a 3 count), chest torso (etc.) and finally your head and neck.
* Rub your hands together as you would to warm them after coming inside from the cold.
* Sway back and forth and slowly wave your arms as if you were leading an orchestra in a lullaby.

Comment What you have been doing is the first step in briefly stimulating the SNS. You are creating a "mini-stress" with this procedure, so that you can tolerate "safe levels." This addition will help you prepare for Relaxation Breathing procedures that follow.

RELAXATION BREATHING
(PARADOX OF CONTROLLING BREATHING
TO DEVELOP UNCONTROLLED BREATHING)

Energy conservation and healing are synonymous with a properly functioning PSNS. Notice that as we practice deep breathing, the PSNS is challenged. In a healthy situation, deep breathing temporarily diminishes the SNS, resulting in an enlarging[*] Accordion Reserve©. However, for many individuals who have a weakened PSNS, the SNS is first stimulated by breathing exercises because the muscle movement is a physical stress, much like an exercise program. The PSNS then responds secondarily, and again we are expanding our Body Tolerance level. With practice, over time, PSNS gradually gains and maintains strength, and the Accordion Reserve© remains expanded.[**]

If you are used to breathing only into the upper chest, the following exercises may cause some dizziness or hyperventilation. If so, you have not been breathing deeply enough and your system is not used to it. Practice these exercises either sitting or lying down until you have no symptoms that could cause you to lose your balance. Later, practice them while standing, sitting or walking so you can incorporate them into your daily life.

PROCEDURE

* I place one hand on my diaphragm and the other on my lower abdomen.

---

[*] Notice that we have highlighted the tense of certain words when relating the size and movement of the Accordion; "**ed**" refers to the size as in "expanded," whereas "**ing**" refers to movement, as in "expanding."
[**] See above comment about "ed" and "ing."

* As I inhale slowly through my nose, I force my lower abdomen to swell like a balloon.
* As I slowly breathe out through my mouth, I drop my jaw and shoulders.

While useful for everyone, the procedure above is especially helpful for the chronically ill and over-achievers (executives, leaders and others who are accustomed to being in control).

♪♪♪♪♪

Like many patients with environmentally triggered problems and many high achievers, I had difficulty with even this simple relaxation breathing exercise so I modified it as follows:

♪♪♪♪♪

PROCEDURE FOR INHALING

* Simultaneously visualizing my whole body (not just my diaphragm) as the balloon, I slowly breathe in through my nose.
* I force out my lower abdomen, keeping my diaphragm and lower abdomen filled with air.
* I fill my body with oxygen, simultaneously expanding my chest, back and shoulders.
* I bring oxygen up through my neck, blowing up my cheeks as I fill them with air.
* Once my body is forced out or filled up, I don't let my abdomen or diaphragm collapse.
* My whole body is the balloon.
* I hold my breath for a count of 3 with my cheeks blown up.

Note to Beginners: Your body frequently begins to relax before the feeling penetrates your conscious mind. By thinking "I feel..." your conscious mind eventually catches up with your body and you learn to listen.

PROCEDURE FOR RELAXING AS YOU EXHALE

* I drop my jaw and shoulders as I slowly breathe out the poisons and tensions through my mouth.
* I feel my body relaxing and growing limp.
* Once I am completely done exhaling, I yawn (force a yawn if necessary).
* Again I drop my jaw and shoulders and feel relaxed.

You will find it very difficult to lock your diaphragm when you drop your jaw to force the yawn. With enough practice your body will automatically yawn whenever you do deep breathing exercises. Yawning is one of nature's ways of relaxing.

INTRODUCTION TO OUR FORM OF MEDITATION

Preparations Lie down in a quiet comfortable place on an exercise mat, mattress or floor. Throughout these instructions "mat" will refer to the flat surface you use. Loosen any tight clothing. Place your neck in a neutral comfortable position. Close your eyes to shut out visual distractions.

* Practice "Relaxation Breathing" 3 times, including the following two instructions.
* "Listen" to your body.
* Think, "I feel relaxed" as you concentrate on the sensations in your body.

INTRODUCTION TO IMAGERY

Imagery is a sensation of an image. Everyone has heard the expression "Mental Image." Most often we think of that image as a visual one. But, in fact, you can also experience a mental image associated with sound, taste, touch or smell. As you proceed through the chapters, you will explore the power and beauty of imagery.

A WORD ABOUT VISUALIZATION

Visualization is a technique to protect the PSNS and reduce the over-stimulation of the SNS, which is directly involved with distress, as Chapter 6 describes "fright, then flight or fight."

Unlike lower kingdom animals that relax the minute the danger has passed, we retain the memory of the cause of the tension. Both negative and positive thoughts distract us from any learning process (negative reinforcements). **Instead of concentrating on techniques, we use visualization as a way of avoiding distractions.** As you follow the chapters, notice how numerous images and variations apply to different procedures. Mix and match them as they suit you. Until your own insights emerge, use those of patients we cite[2] or ours.

SUMMARY
PLAYING THE ACCORDION RESERVE©

Necessary to your healing is the introduction of a breathing system that concentrates on balancing the SNS with the PSNS. Your own system will evolve as you practice, using our guidelines and developing your own variations.

Practice several times, always three breaths in a set. "Listen" to your breathing between sets. Be consistent. The consistent repetition in a pattern of three develops a patterned response. In time you will develop automatic uncontrolled diaphragmatic breathing.

What follows is a culmination of what you learned in this chapter. Natalie tells us how the techniques apply to her and to others:

♫♫♫♫♫

I find that visualizing and adding physical movement to my visualization increases the effectiveness of my breathing and prepares me for Meditation/Relaxation Healing.

When I first wake up while still lying on my bed, I stimulate my nerve endings by tapping as described above. I stretch both my arms perpendicular to the ceiling, the palms of my hands facing each other about six inches apart.

As I practice Relaxation Breathing three times (see above), I visualize playing an accordion. As I breathe in, I pull my hands apart as far as possible, as if I were expanding the bellows of the accordion, at the same time visualizing expanding my lungs.

As I breathe out, I stretch, pulling my hands together, visualizing playing the music as I visualize exhaling poisons from my lungs.

In subsequent chapters you will be able to see how I use additional visual, vocal, physical and spiritual techniques culminating in the Meditation/Relaxation Healing and completing the musical analogy.

VARIATIONS

Alan added a new concept – incorporating an exercise ball (like a large globe about 24 inches in diameter). Circling the ball, he stretches his arms over his head, moving his torso to the left as he breathes in and holds. Then he slowly breathes out as he stretches to the right (still holding the ball). His second breath begins to the right and his third begins toward the left. (I expanded on Alan's concept by visualizing holding a hula-hoop.)

"Philip" (not his real name) amended my procedure. First he stretches his hands out as I do, visualizing the accordion opening to full breadth. Then he swings his arms back together as if he were making a halo over his head, locking his fingers, palms facing the ceiling, pushing his shoulders backward and stretching his chest muscles and expanding his lungs.

Depending on our moods, we practice the techniques several times a day, using variations of our own ideas and ideas from patients who are always finding new ways.

It is effective if you use music in any dimension — sing, hum, play a recording, listen to the radio, etc. To stimulate our energy field, we precede our exercises by acting out the role of an orchestra leader, physically when possible, imaginatively when not.

Patients frequently prefer to begin practicing our procedure first for a few times and then move on to their own variation using their creativity.
♫♫♫♫

Now you are ready for PHASE II, in which you will add Body Awareness to your breathing.

---

[1] "Bioelectricity," 15th Annual International Symposium on Man and His Environment, sponsored by AAEM and the American Environmental Health Foundation, Dallas, TX.
[2] Cited by permission.

8

BODY AWARENESS
- Phase II -
Your Awakening

Prologue

♪♪♪♪

<u>Body Awareness — New Concepts</u> An explanation is in order for readers of my previous books. I have always used the term Body Awareness to distinguish between different simultaneous sensations: one cold, one warm foot; one heavy, one light hand; one loose, one tense arm, etc.

I have also described Body Awareness for the sensation when you are in a relaxed state. I called the total sensation "The Feeling."

As Alan developed his own skills of Body Awareness with my guidance, he told me he preferred to change my term "The Feeling" to "The Awakening." To him the sensation was a flash back to infancy. He told me that as a pediatrician he associated the feeling with the moment when infants "tune in" to their own "Feeling" of the world.

♪♪♪♪

DEFINITIONS AS USED IN THIS BOOK

Body Awareness describes your ability to distinguish sensations in different areas of your body at the same time.

"The Awakening" describes the overall relaxed sensation that envelops you from head to toe. In other words, as you shall see, Body Awareness is a prerequisite to experiencing Your Awakening.

To be "*Grounded*" is the state when you experience the quiet and peaceful flow of energy from the ground through the soles of your feet, through the top of your head and beyond, then returning along the same path. The sensation is like feeling your feet anchored in soil. You will recognize that you must experience "The Awakening" in order to be grounded.

For Aches, Pains and Other Symptoms Until you learn to ground yourself, Body Awareness – "listening" to your body – is more an exercise of learning to feel your body. As you progress you will be able to listen and hear your vibrations.

Body Awareness is essential to healing.

By becoming aware of your body sensations you develop a warning signal to slow down or even stop a reaction before it manifests itself. Why wait until pain becomes unbearable? Body Awareness is even more important for chronic than for acute reactions. However, first sense your unique Body Awareness.

♪♪♪♪

My Negative Body Awareness Experience

In 1969, because we could find no anesthesia I could tolerate, my allergist, Dr. Eloise Kailin, sent me to a hypnotist to prepare me for extensive dental work. The process was counterproductive because I had trouble understanding his accent. Also, he instructed me to direct warmth to my limbs, but I felt only cold. I became frustrated and experienced stress rather than relaxation – the state necessary for a self-induced anesthetized state.

Turning a Negative into a Positive Thanks to my mentor, Dr. James C. Cox, I was able to change my negative experience into the positive program presented in this book. Under Dr. Cox's tutelage I studied with many teachers, psychiatrists, psychologists and therapists of massage, dance, theater and movement. From each energy modality and especially from Dr. Cox's lessons, I pieced together a program suited to my own Body Awareness.

I learned that it is inaccurate to assume that everyone in a relaxed state experiences the same sensations. Therefore, even if you have experienced a modality guiding you to a specific sensation, you may find your body sensations keep changing and reaching greater depths.

My awareness continually changes. During my meditative state, my insights take me into new heights. So will yours as you progress.

♪♪♪♪♪

Note to Beginners Before you begin to practice PHASE II, read the entire chapter for a description of the process and an understanding of the goal of Body Awareness. A second or third reading is sometimes required to motivate beginners to practice. Proceed at your own pace.

Meditation/Relaxation Healing PRACTICE (rather than "try") the exercises! ("Practice" involves an active, balanced commitment to learn!) Furthermore, Patience is the key to successful relaxation healing! High expectations and goal setting undermine your practice experiences. For a change of pace, liberate yourself as you practice. Savor the pleasure and freedom of relaxation.

Once you have reached total relaxation, the process can be as relaxing as sedatives – without side effects. Just as a starter, Meditation/Relaxation Healing has been known to prevent blistering from burns and speed recovery of open wounds and broken bones.

HOW TO ACHIEVE THE RELAXED FEELING (REVISITED)

Preparations The word "mat" refers to an exercise mat or any soft, flat surface providing padding on the floor.

61

* Lie down in a quiet comfortable place on a mat. Loosen any tight clothing.
* Place your neck in a neutral, comfortable position.
* Close your eyes to shut out visual distractions.
* Practice "Relaxation Breathing" 3 times (see Chapter 7).

PROGRESSIVE MUSCLE RELAXATION AND Body Awareness

<u>Body Awareness - First Encounters</u> Practice learning the following progressive muscle relaxation technique, as you introduce music by thinking it, singing it or listening to a recording:

* Listen and recognize the early stage of your energy sensations.
* Acquire a new vocabulary of more precise words to describe your energy.
* Pinpoint sensations you feel when you are relaxed.

PROCEDURE

During this exercise with your right leg, keep your left leg straight and relaxed on the mat. Later you will exercise the left leg using the same instructions.

Practice each exercise three times to begin developing a conditional response.

1. Stretch Your Right Leg

* Keep your heel touching the mat. Push your heel away from your head. Pull your toes toward you. Tighten your leg.
* Feel tension (but not pain) moving up through the calf, behind the knee and up to your buttocks.
* Hold this position to the count of 3.

* Release the tension very, very slowly to avoid straining your muscles.
* Let your leg go limp. Sense your heel and toes relaxing as they return to the resting position.
* Practice three times, gradually increasing the holding position to the count of 3.

2. Synchronize Your Breathing and Leg Stretching (This is in the first step of uniting the six phases of Parts III and IV.)

Repeat the leg stretch simultaneously with Relaxation Breathing, blowing up your whole body as if it were a balloon (see Relaxation Breathing in Chapter 7). Slowly inhale through your nose as you tense your leg. Keeping your heel on the mat, as you push your heel away from your head, pull your toes toward your head.

* Hold your breath as you maintain leg tension.
* Slowly exhale through your mouth as you slowly release the leg tension.
* Sense the change as you pause.
* Slowly increase your lung capacity, counting to 3 twice, then to 3 three times, etc. to coincide with your breathing pattern.

EMPHASIS: Breathe in as you tense up, hold your breath during the tension; breathe out when you relax. Remember to relax your muscles slowly to avoid strain. Make a mental note of the feeling of being relaxed, another technique of listening to your body.

3. Compare Your Legs

* This time as you tense your right leg with synchronized breathing, compare the feeling in your right leg with that in your left leg.
* While holding your breath focus on a distinct difference between the tensed right leg and the relaxed left.

* Concentrate and feel the difference between your legs, tensed and relaxed.
* Breathe out slowly and relax, releasing the tension in your leg slowly to avoid straining your muscles.
* Become aware of your legs. Compare them. How do they feel? Does one leg feel better than the other? In what way? How do they feel on the mat?
* Make a mental note of any sensations you have in your legs.

EMPHASIS: Focus on different sensations between your tensed leg and untensed leg.

* Monitor your Sensations.
* Repeat the "Compare Your Legs" exercise two more times with the right leg to reinforce the pattern of three.
* Savor the evolving sense of **Body Awareness** (the feeling of your **Relaxed State**) that occurs in your tensed right leg as it approaches and then becomes more relaxed than your untensed left leg.

EMPHASIS: Focus on the improved feeling of relaxation in the tensed leg after it has been stretched and let go.

Use the Experience It is now time to name your sensation of relaxation. Do you feel warm or cool, heavy or light? Does your right leg feel longer or shorter? Does it feel as if it is sinking or floating? Does it feel weightless or have a tingling sensation? Is it energized? Ignore the word "relaxed" and develop a new, very personal language to define your relaxed state. Be very specific. Later, using the names will help reproduce relaxation.

The above are sensations people have experienced. You may feel a combination of these or none of them. You may also experience different sensations each time you practice. Let your imagination flow. That is part of the experience. Become creative with your description, like the man who reported that his legs felt like "huge watermelons," people who feel they are swimming in a bowl of Jell-O™ or "Philip", who describes himself as "amorphous."

NOTE You may also become aware of an emotional feeling – peaceful, calm, etc., but for now concentrate on the physical sensations.

EMPHASIS: Draw on your own experiences.

A Positive Attitude Maintain your spirit. Because yours is a very personal perception, your initial awareness may be slow or fast. As you practice day-to-day, your personal encounters will also change in intensity and duration. Each day's experience is unique. Be prepared for unexpected variations.

Some people who have benefited most from this process required a lengthy time before they generated awareness of changes in their body. Now they can relax so completely that they anesthetize themselves, stop bleeding or speed up the healing of wounds, etc. Follow the instructions and complete the exercise. You will soon notice a change.

4. Balance Your Legs

*   <u>Left Leg</u> Repeat the *PROCEDURE* using instructions for your right leg (see above 1, 2 and 3).
*   <u>Both Legs</u> Now tighten both legs at the same time, using synchronized breathing.
*   <u>Compare the feeling in your legs</u> to your memory of your initial sensations. Recall the continuing changes in sensations.

♪♪♪♪♪

Now that you have learned the first steps of PHASE II, here is an inspiration for you to practice, perfect and advance to the next steps.

65

At one time I had frequent bouts of temporary partial paralysis on my left side — I could move neither my arm nor my leg. Beginning with Step 1 of Meditation/Relaxation Healing, I was able to relax my right foot and right leg. Using imagery along with the subsequent steps enabled me to shorten periods of paralysis.

At first the procedure was useful because I could release severe cramps in my right leg and right arm and frequently other parts of my body. After a long time I reached a point where I could prevent paralysis.

Have you ever had a "toothache" in your leg? Yes, it sounds funny, but sometimes cramping in my legs was so intense it felt like a toothache. When I had that feeling, I was able to relieve the pain. At this point I can usually ward off pain or paralysis by using Meditation/Relaxation Healing.

♫♫♫♫

<u>Body Awareness Revisited</u> With practice, concentrating on your right stretched leg and comparing it with your left relaxed leg enables you to pinpoint a precise site of tension in your body. Practice continues by applying the same exercise to other body parts such as your:

* Arms (fists, then forearms, then upper arms)
* Jaw (gnashing your teeth together and jutting your jaw forward)
* Face (squinting your eyes closed, wrinkling your nose, sticking out your tongue)
* Torso (shrugging shoulders, tensing pelvic and sphincter muscles)
* Create your own variations on this theme

Repeated experiences prepare you to expand the relaxation technique to include tensing your entire body, then relaxing it, in sequence. Next, you can synchronize tensing-relaxing with the breathing-relaxing exercise.

This fundamental sensation (tension contrasting with relaxation) enhances your **Body Awareness** and leads to **Meditation/Relaxation Healing.** The applications of this procedure are virtually infinite. Undoubtedly you will find your own personal situations. For example:

* Grinding your teeth (bruxism) can be reduced or eliminated.
* Constipation or diarrhea resulting from chemical exposure may improve.
* Urinary frequency may be decreased.
* Muscle aches and pain may be negated.

Abbreviated Instructions Before beginning to practice the entire PHASE II *PROCEDURES,* copy the following instructions onto a 3" by 5" card to keep close at hand beside your bed or tape them on a recorder, allowing time to respond to the instructions.

PROCEDURE

* Lie down; close eyes; compare legs.
* Inhale for tensing, hold breath during the tension and exhale for relaxing.
* Check body sensations between steps.
* Tighten and relax in sequence:
            -right leg, left leg, both legs;
            -right arm, left arm, both arms;
            -jaws, face, head, neck;
            -upper and lower torso;
            -whole body at one time.

The Awakening

Enjoy the relaxed state. Be aware of your body, your breathing and your surroundings. You deserve the feeling of well-being that now floods throughout. It may well be your first awareness of the sensation of your individual energy flow.

<u>The Awakening</u> You will know when you experience a new sensation that we call "The Awakening." No one can describe it for you. It's a little like falling in love. When it happens, you will know.

Tuning into Your Awakening *and Naming It* To help you recognize **Your Awakening**, as you lie on the mat, become aware of your total sensations and how your arms and legs (and other body parts) feel – if you can feel them at all. Note the sensation of which you are most aware and most enjoy. Give **Your Awakening** a name. For example, you might call it "weightless," "floating," "heaviness," "tingling," "energizing" or perhaps "vacuum."

We were born with the feeling, awareness, awakening or you name it. As negatives entered our consciousness as toddlers, we blocked our feelings. However, they remained in our subconscious. These exercises can restore the memory of your early sensations.

<u>Key Words - "I feel"</u> If you keep repeating "I feel," you are programming or conditioning your **Mind/body/soul/spirit** to recall the memory and then use the conditioned memory for relaxing.

Use your choice of the name freely, substituting it whenever you read the words **"The Awakening."** This new language is a way for you to communicate with your own body: "I feel weightless," or "I feel energized," or "I feel tingling," or "I feel heavy" or whatever your feeling happens to be. This is the beginning of the conditioning process to induce rapid whole body relaxation.

SHORTCUT *TO* The Awakening

We will refer to this procedure many more times throughout the book. It is essential that you know how to use the **SHORTCUT** as a means of instantaneous relaxation. The more often you use it, the more it becomes a habit.

* Simultaneously slowly take a deep breath, tighten your entire body; tense your legs as you pull your toes toward

68

your head; make fists while tensing your arms and shoulders; bite down on an imaginary pencil; tense your face, head and neck; and tighten muscles in your torso, back, abdomen, pelvis and buttocks.

* Hold this tension as you hold your breath.
* Breathe out very slowly.
* Let your entire body go limp.
* Keep repeating, "My Mind/body/soul/spirit merge into a unity as I feel The Awakening" — (use the name you call Your Awakening). Repeat three times.
* Practice the **SHORTCUT** in a sitting position at home so you can use it in your car (before you start the engine) and other places where you have to be seated.

Be sure you are describing your own feeling. Don't adopt labels you may have heard others use to describe their relaxed feeling. Use the word or expression that best describes what you feel in your relaxed state. Remember: Draw on Your Own Experiences. The more you practice, the more your feelings will change. Be sure you understand how to use this **SHORTCUT** to The Awakening because we will refer to this procedure throughout the book.

♫♫♫♫

Recall playing the Accordion Reserve© in the last paragraph of Chapter 7: "Breath of Health," when I physically and visually act out playing the accordion, so the full impact of the exercise penetrates my body.

Now build on that exercise by including Your Awakening.
♫♫♫♫

Example Visually and physically keep repeating what your body is feeling as you breathe out, pushing the accordion closed. Concentrate on Your Awakening as you visualize collapsing the accordion, generating music as you exhale toxins from your lungs with a "hah" sound. When you are not alone you may sound "hah" very quietly, even imperceptibly. When alone give the "hah" sound full voice.

SUMMARY

Body Awareness is a sensation you have probably felt in your lifetime but never realized what it was. For some it is a vibration, a tingling or a pulsation. Notice that this sensation is a primitive touch or sound image. Playing the Accordion is at first a visual image, but by combining it with your Body Awareness, you embellish the imagery. You can also include a physical sound like a sustained "hah" to the image. As you vibrate from the sound and movement of your arms, the imagery becomes very powerful and positively reinforces your experience. The imagery may remind you of a time when you were at a concert, and the band played a melody with a harmony and a rhythm that gave you "shivers" or "goose bumps." That is Your Awakening.

As you continue, you will see how we tie up lessons for all chapters so you can develop your own unique program. You are now ready to move on to PHASE III – "Conditioning."

9

CONDITIONING
- Phase III -
Building or Changing Patterns

Prologue

The following six paragraphs were originally written to introduce conditioning theory to the novice. What follows, however, also benefits professionals well versed in conditioning techniques. Unique to this discussion is the melding of the Accordion Reserve© with standard procedures. We have found that the ultimate synthesis results in a powerful tool to expand personal energy.

Conditioning In psychology, conditioning is a process whereby a stimulus — feeling, object or situation — begins to elicit a certain response that differs from the usual or normal response to that stimulus. In other words, if you normally react in a certain way to a particular substance, you can train yourself to react in the same way to a different stimulus by continuously associating the one with the other. Conditioning is a learned behavior.

Deconditioning We must also consider the processes of altering conditioned patterns or deconditioning responses. The difference between conditioned and deconditioned responses will be demonstrated below.

Research Pavlov conducted the best-known research in conditioning. Before he fed research dogs, he rang a bell. The dogs were soon conditioned to salivate at the sound of the bell, even in the absence of food. In *Time Magazine*, Oxford scientist Matt Ridley[1] wrote about Pavlov's experiment: "...we know how the brain changes: by the real-time expression of 17 genes, known as the CREB genes...genes allow the human mind to learn, remember, imitate, and

71

imprint language, absorb culture, and express instincts. Genes are not puppet masters or blueprints, nor are they just the carriers of heredity. They are active during life; they switch one another on and off; they respond to the environment." The complex interaction of genes and environment (external and internal) may have multiple mechanisms that induce conditioning.

Need for Positive Thoughts For the conditioning process to work in stress reduction, you must be totally convinced you have the ability to improve your physical condition by your thoughts. Negative thoughts often impede the process and ironically prove that your thoughts affect your body. Only you can make the choice as to whether your thoughts have a positive or negative effect on your well-being.

Harmful Negative Thoughts The idea is well established that thoughts affect the body. We were born with the ability to use our thoughts positively, but often use them negatively. Knowing that thoughts affect your body will convince you of the importance of your beliefs, attitudes and commonly used expressions. Think of a traumatic exposure or experience and notice how you tense up. Think of sucking a lemon and you salivate.

Clinical experience suggests that tensions can be transmitted to any area of one's anatomy. For example, if he has underlying pathophysiologic preconditioning, an infant can refer tension to his skin, resulting in eczema, or to his stomach in the form of colic. In an adult, examples of negative transmission are a "tension headache" and "butterflies in the stomach."

Turning Negatives into Positives Just as negative thoughts can cause headaches, positive thoughts can erase them. Working from this premise, we have developed the following conditioning process to reinforce positive thoughts by repetition. But first practice the following short example:

* Take three deep breaths and relax as you learned in Chapter 7.
* Sense how your body feels.
* Think of a happy, pleasant experience.
* Note the changes that occur in your body.
* Note especially where the relaxation is apparent.
* Now shift your thoughts to a very stressful situation.
* Note the changes caused simply by your thoughts.
* If negative thoughts can cause symptoms, is it not logical that positive thoughts erase them?

Pattern of Repetition Conditioning is most effective with a pattern of repetition. In PHASE I, we suggested repeating each step three times. In Chapter 7 you learned Relaxation Breathing, practicing three times to set a pattern of repetition. You followed the pattern three times, synchronizing your breathing with stretching. It was suggested that if it is necessary to repeat, do so in a pattern of threes.

♪♪♪♪

For the most effective conditioning, I have found the greatest success in a consistent pattern. Alan prefers concluding some practice sessions by counting from one to ten. Some patients prefer counting back from three to one. If you too have been conditioned in other modalities with other counts, do what suits you best in as consistent a pattern as possible.

♪♪♪♪

Synchronizing Your Breathing with Positive Thoughts
You are a Master of the SHORTCUT. You are experienced at synchronizing two body functions – breathing and muscle tension. The sensation – "The Awakening" – is your memory of that pleasurable experience. You will now learn to condition yourself - synchronizing

your body and mind, for which you have a name and which we call The Awakening. Please substitute your personalized expression.

Ever-changing Cycle Before you begin, remember that each time you practice, you may experience the same or different sensations; as a result you will experience varying improvements in your conditioning. Note: You can use varying fluctuations as a sign of your changing Accordion Reserve©.

Mind/body/soul/spirit Awareness Conditioning consists of the SHORTCUT, followed by Relaxation Breathing exercises synchronized to your positive thoughts. You breathe in as you tense and breathe out as you relax, just as you did in PHASE I (Chapter 7).

PROCEDURE

* Establish your relaxation using the SHORTCUT (Chapter 8).
* Practice Diaphragmatic Breathing and Synchronized Breathing with Muscle Tension and Stretching.
* Re-experience Your Awakening.

From this point on, whenever you see the words "The Awakening," use the term that most accurately describes Your Awakening — weightless, heavy, tingling, etc.

* I slowly breathe in oxygen, silently counting to three as I say or just think, "I feel The Awakening."
* I hold my breath and focus on feeling and experiencing The Awakening.
* I breathe out slowly, savoring the beauty of The Awakening, repeating phrases like "I Relax with The Awakening," "The Awakening is Beautiful." (At the same time, if you happen to remember a smell, taste, touch, sound or a visual experience as you relax, add it to your thoughts and phrases. This is imagery.)
* Draw on your pleasurable experiences.

74

* To follow the pattern of three, repeat the sequence twice more.
* Conclude your practice session with a formula like, "When I count back from three to zero, I am alert and so relaxed that my Mind/body/soul/spirit has absorbed The Awakening, has recorded the procedure and conditioned me to reproduce The Awakening whenever my body feels tense."

Emphasis: Synchronizing a pleasurable experience with thoughts about the sensation will ultimately condition you. *Be creative! Be unique!* Recall that in PHASE I, you associated exhaling with relaxing your muscles. Now you are associating the delightful sensation of The Awakening with *breathing* (a body function) *and your positive thoughts* (a mind function). In time, just focusing on the thoughts will allow you to revisit the experience and the relaxation that is associated with it. That is *conditioning* in a positive, constructive use of the ideomotor principle.

At some stage of your experience with PHASE III, you will be able to create your own conditioned SHORTCUT, just as you did with PHASE II. At this level of expertise, relaxation is almost automatic. For example:

PROCEDURE

* Breathe in Deeply....
* Breathe out Slowly as You:
    * Think "one"
      I feel The Awakening
    * Think "two"
      I feel The Awakening
    * Think "three"
      I feel The Awakening

Daily practice of the Conditioning Procedure builds your confidence. Confidence builds self-esteem. Self-esteem also builds confidence. This reinforcing cycle allows you to relax even more. Relaxation clears clutter from your mind and eventually you will be able to explore pleasant memories that remind you of The Awakening. In turn, these hidden treasures will induce even greater relaxation.

Joy and exhilaration often flow from these discoveries. Whether you call it a "rush," a "high" or just "euphoria," you will sooner or later experience your personal essence – your spirit and soul. Allow yourself the freedom to uncover your past. It is a remarkable adventure. Add each new encounter to your memory bank. From time to time, you may update The Awakening, incorporating your essence, spirit and soul. Daily progress is usually imperceptible. Yet, suddenly one day you may discover an entirely new tranquility and peace of mind.

From time to time during the day apply the *PROCEDURE* or SHORTCUT for PHASE III during a three-minute period. It is a powerful way to eliminate unnecessary tensions, allowing you to handle stress without jeopardizing your health. Even when confronted by unavoidable stress caused by pollution or negative situations, stress responses can be reduced. When you are relaxed, stressful situations will affect you less.

Instant Relaxation of PHASE III Recall what you have learned so far. PHASE I teaches you Relaxation Breathing. PHASE II teaches you to experience The Awakening. PHASE III teaches you to condition yourself to reach The Awakening. PHASE III is an extension of PHASE II: the time necessary to achieve the relaxed state is virtually nil. You may also discover that you slide back and forth between PHASE II and PHASE III.

Be positive even if relaxation does not come automatically after several practices. Be aware that relaxation is not always automatic, even after you have achieved it before and have learned automatic conditioning. After all, we are all individuals and many factors influence our ability to relax, especially those factors that influence the Accordion Reserve©. The reserve itself influences relaxation, just as relaxation influences reserve.

It is ironic that persons who do not have extra time to practice relaxation techniques are the ones who need it most because they are burdened with stress. It is worth taking time now to achieve **PHASE III** because in the long run it will improve your health and actually save you time. For example, you can use **PHASE III CONDITIONING** to improve your sleep. Your sleep will be more restful; therefore you will require less sleep, wake up more refreshed and have more energy. Thus, you have expanded your **Accordion Reserve**©.

ALAN'S THOUGHTS ON CONDITIONING

♫♫♫♫♫

I have found that another feature of the conditioning technique for me is the opportunity to reread the above 3 procedures of Mind/body/soul/spirit awareness. While Natalie has worked with and taught RELAXATION for years, I still regard myself as a relative novice. In fact, we are all perpetual students.

From time to time, I have found that My Awakening is less relaxing than it used to be. Sometimes images get stale and can be refreshed or images that were once useful but discarded can be recycled. The above paragraphs are, for me, a way of super-charging my technique.

Learning a New Skill Conditioning may appear to be a new exercise for you, but in fact, any time you learn a new skill you are conditioning yourself. An example of a function you usually take for granted is bodily elimination. For a toddler, though, learning bowel control is a challenging experience and the anxiety it generates sometimes remains in the adult subconscious. Becoming potty trained without traumas, however, is a simple exercise in effective conditioning. I have included in this chapter my potty training technique for parents.

The demonstration includes five points: introducing a concept, repeating the concept, reinforcing the concept with a message, building success

77

through repetition and reward and finally a serial refinement of the concept.

Natalie's conditioning technique and mine are analogous. So even before we met, we were following a common path until our Guiding Force brought us together to unite our core of energy work and create the Accordion Reserve©.

♫♫♫♫♫

POTTY TRAINING

Potty training is a skill a child can gradually acquire at the parents' discretion (approximately 18 to 24 months). The basic concept is that there is a time and a place for everything — there is a right time and a right place to go to the potty. When the child learns that step, the rest becomes an enhancement of the basic process.

CAUTIONS: Control Issues Because potty training is such a control issue, the object is to have both child and parent in control of the same situation at the same time. So avoid the question: "Do you want to go to the potty?" This question gives the child control.

Avoiding Anxiety Issues

1. The potty seat should be a separate floor model rather than attached to the toilet during the target phases. Some toddlers may develop the fear of falling into the toilet.

2. Flushing the toilet in the presence of the youngster can create several anxieties depending on the timing. If the potty is attached to the toilet and the child is sitting on it, he may perceive that he will be flushed away. If the stool is dumped in the toilet after a diaper change or after successful elimination in the potty-chair, the darling may perceive that "his creation" is being thrown away. This feeling undermines the otherwise successful accomplishment.

3. Prior to the third stage of potty training, refrain from removing the toddler's diaper during the hide and seek game described below.

This additional process increases stress since two actions would have to be learned simultaneously.

Patterning Issues Observe for a pattern of the child's movements. Stools usually follow a toddler's meal. If you recognize his pattern, then you begin the program to coincide with the expected pattern.

TARGET PRACTICE PROCEDURE

Refer to **Figure 9-1** to follow the three-step process of Conditioning.

Step 1.

* The outer ring on the target represents the right time and the right place as it links the bathroom to making a bowel movement.
* In the bathroom place a potty-chair and a toy friend (like a teddy bear) sitting on the potty.
* Play a game of hide and seek throughout your living space to go looking for the teddy bear.
* When the child's friend is eventually found, comment on how comfortable teddy is on the potty-chair.
* Always end up in the bathroom at the time that the toddler is ready to make a poop.
* Play the game daily or more often if the toddler has a more frequent stool pattern.
* If the child winds up playing in the bathroom and pooping in his diaper, then you say, "Look at that! That's wonderful! You made in your diaper in the bathroom. Let's go and change your diaper!"
* Continue to play the game, always calling attention to the fact that the child has pooped in his diaper while he was in the bathroom.
* That message begins to link the time and the place with the action.

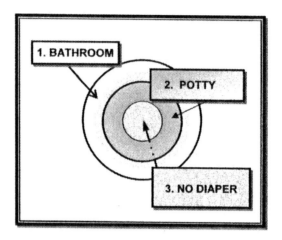

> Figure 9-1. Target Practice for Potty Training. Toddler should be in the Right Place at the Right Time. Settings for Right Place are sequentially more specific and refining.

<u>*Comment*</u> Please note the potty is always in the bathroom while the game is being played. In STEP 1 however, avoid suggesting that the youngster sit on the potty-chair. If he sits down on the potty that is fine, but it is not to be promoted.

Step 2.

Having successfully completed STEP 1 (toddler consistently poops in the diaper while in the bathroom), the next inner ring on the target makes one change only: substituting the potty-chair for the bathroom itself as "the place." Timing remains the same. In STEP 1, the youngster has observed his friend feeling comfortable in the potty-chair. (Remember: do not remove the diaper at this stage.)

* Encourage the child to sit on the potty-chair while he plays a game or reads a book to his toy friend.
* If the child succeeds by pooping in his diaper while sitting on the potty, say, "Look at that! You made in the

diaper while you sat on the potty seat. That's wonderful! Let's go change your diaper."
* Repeat the process many times as you did with the first ring.

Step 3.

The third step (bull's-eye) repeats the game. The only change at this stage: playing the game with the diaper off. Nonchalantly, remove the diaper prior to the start of hide and seek (later on, you could remove it on entering the bathroom).

* Comment on the diaper being off after the success has occurred.
* Applaud "the little one's terrific accomplishment."

Comment Potty training is a three-step process of conditioning that requires only one learning linkage: there is a right time and a right place. Once that is accomplished everything else follows. Successful conditioning requires positive encouragement or reinforcement.

Reinforcement

* **Positive Reinforcement** is a reward with encouraging words, applause or small material gestures. Giving a reward every time is called **Continuous Positive Reinforcement**. The emotion of joy or exhilaration results from positive reinforcement.
* **Intermittent Positive Reinforcement** means <u>sometimes</u> providing rewards, but <u>not every time,</u> after the desired behavior is repeated and reinforced.
* **Negative Reinforcement** is a discouraging action that is applied after a specific behavior. Refusing to give attention, denying eye contact, and a firm squeeze or tap on the hand are some examples. Sadness, guilt, anger, frustration or embarrassment often result from or contribute to negative reinforcement.

* Conflicts and control issues are negative reinforcement and discourage the conditioning process.

* Intermittent Reinforcement – either positive or negative – is more powerful than Continuous Reinforcement of either type.

* <u>Inconsistent</u> response to a behavior is equivalent to Intermittent Reinforcement.

* <u>If you want to discourage a behavior, you must provide Continuous Negative Reinforcement</u>.

* If you are inconsistent in providing Negative Reinforcement or you are sometimes involved in conflicts and control issues, you are more strongly reinforcing an undesirable behavior or discouraging a desirable behavior.

♫♫♫♫♫

Notice the three steps are similar to Natalie's conditioning process presented in PHASES I, II and III. It is the same process Pavlov demonstrated when he conditioned dogs to salivate at the sound of a bell, even in the absence of food. My system of potty training is just one example of early childhood conditioning used to prevent lifetime stresses that can contribute to system responses like constipation. The same process can be applied to many areas of discipline and training of children. To put it succinctly, early childhood conditioning can begin the process of building the Accordion Reserve©.

Spontaneous Deconditioning

After chemical, emotional or physical traumas, de-conditioning is the process of relieving all aspects of Mind/body/soul/spirit tensions. Dreams are one form of spontaneous deconditioning. An example follows of one such life-changing event, which helped me but for some people resulted in major distress.

On July 20, 1995, Natalie and I did not know each other. I did not know anything about the wonderful techniques you are currently learning. On that day, five beautiful people were murdered in my neighborhood. Four of them were my friends. They were David, Andrea, Sherry and Alyse Goff. I was not emotionally prepared for these brutal acts of violence. Is anybody? Had I learned and practiced the techniques you read today, I believe I would have been better prepared. But sometimes an inner strength (soul/spirit) helps one cope. And so I share with you an excerpt from an essay I wrote on July 22, 1995 to help me decondition the ordeal.

I did not know it at the time, but I was spontaneously practicing Natalie's process of soul-searching. I can't explain why, but I sat down at my computer and poured out my grief. In the manner of stream of consciousness, the following is an excerpt from what I wrote about the violence. I include it as a memorial to the murdered Goffs.

"...I shiver and shake. It is an explosion inside. It is erupting. My tears flow like lava, hot and furious. When will my emotions ever stop? I am afraid they will never stop - never! I AM HUMAN!

"I seek to control my emotions. I cannot. The feelings are inside.

"They always were. But they never came out. What words can I use to tell what agony is inside of me? I sit, I shake. The violence is erupting as I type. The lava flows. The fears, the screams, the inner violence flows in fury.

"I shake some more. I have always done this - this shaking - when I am scared, nervous or have to relate. I am an inside person. I could never fully share. Why not? I never learned how. I am shaking, crying, erupting again. I am having a temper tantrum. I want to scream and shout and hit and bang and throw things. I want to be violent. I am furious.

"I have been afraid to let it out. I am afraid of what I can do with my own violence. I swing and hit, rant and rave. I can hurt with my hands. I can hurt with my words. I can cause pain. I can be brutal. I can be violent. I am human.

"I am a little boy - crying and scared. There are monsters somewhere. I am shaking. I am terrorized. I keep seeing my friends' beautiful, smiling faces. But they are not smiling. They are shocked, horrified and terrorized by the brutality that their eyes see as they are murdered one by one.

"I am crying violently now - seething, erupting in agony. Pain is pouring out. I can't type fast enough. Tears are coming in torrents now. My nose is dripping like a faucet. The tissues catch the flow. Were it blood, I would be dying. But I cannot die. I must live and move on.

"So what do we do with them? Ignore them? Often! Act out on them? OH, YES! We have temper tantrums. We scream, we yell, we throw, we hit, we curse, we break, we seek to control, we destroy, we abuse, we harass, we dominate, we rape, we shoot, we stab, we kill, we drink, we smoke, we shoot up, we snort, we overeat, we vomit..."

Deconditioning — Violence Revisited As I reread this passage, I still feel grief and tears return. The message is incredibly powerful. In order for me to write as I did, I had to let go of all my usual inhibitions regarding emotional expression. Intuitively, it was absolutely necessary for my spiritual safety. As it turns out, the techniques in these chapters help to cast off the inhibitions that prevent us from healing. My spiritual background helped me experience my catharsis. More about that later.

I am writing this section during the Ten Days of Repentance. On the Day of Atonement, which concludes those solemn days, the congregation communally recites a list of sins in a prayer "Vidui." It is repeated throughout the day. Readers familiar with the liturgy will recognize the last sentence of the excerpt above as a rewording of that prayer which I have known since childhood. The list consists of all possible sins knowingly or unknowingly committed during the year.

BEHAVIOR AND "THE TERRIBLE TWO'S"

Because of my catharsis, I could finally personalize my teaching. I never felt comfortable expressing my emotions, yet as a pediatrician I discovered it is necessary to advise parents about when and how children learn to express their emotions.

I realized that children are learning to express their emotions during the developmental stage frequently called the terrible two's. As the explanation evolved, I realized I was again dealing with simple conditioning. I share it now because I believe that if children are conditioned and incorporate it into their souls at age

two, they will be able to process their emotions more effectively. Thus, many complex emotional disturbances that we see in adulthood would be alleviated.
♫♫♫♫♫

Emotional Conditioning The conditioning process is based on stages of language acquisition. Infants first produce simple sounds. Words are then repeated. First, single words are usually names of things. About age 2 simple two-word sentences include words of action. These are usually visible to toddlers. However, emotion words like "angry," "sad," "happy" and "frustrated" do not have a direct visual connection; thus, they may not be learned as quickly as visually-associated words. Nevertheless emotions do exist inside the child's mind. So how do children express them? By physical action of a "temper tantrum," i.e. the "acting out" of internal emotion.

When observing a "temper tantrum," you, the parent or other caregiver, must determine if the toddler is misbehaving or expressing his emotions. More often than not, "temper tantrums" are assumed to be misbehavior, and children are frequently punished for their actions. However, you should recognize a "temper tantrum" for what it truly is – a physical expression of an emotion that he cannot yet verbalize.

An appropriate response is for you to act like a mirror, so that the child can "see" the emotion. Name the behavior you just observed, as if you were in his shoes. Say something like: "You sure look Angry (or other emotion)!" Then complete the interaction by including the following: "Please tell me that you are Angry. I will Listen to you, and then you will feel better." This response is called Empathy – feeling the emotion that someone else senses. When he echoes your words, your attention is his reward. He feels better and gains a positive sense of sharing experiences.

Through repetition, the toddler will associate his "temper tantrum" action with the "visualized" emotion, which you named for him. This is classic conditioning at its best. Later on, as the child grows older, he will be able to discover why he feels the emotion that he has verbalized. The "why" is the third step in the conditioning process.

Always include a choice of behavior as is appropriate in child discipline: "You may choose to continue yelling and screaming. Do it somewhere else." Offer the consequence of choosing the alternate behavior: "I will not listen to you or pay attention to you while you continue your 'temper tantrum,' and you may continue to feel uncomfortable. However, when you change your mind about telling me, I will still listen to you."

Finally, set limits on the alternative behavior, which is also an appropriate discipline technique. These limits are:

1) Do not destroy property.
2) Do not hurt anyone else.
3) Do not hurt yourself.

Conditioning results from consistently repeating mirrored behavior: encouraging the toddler to verbalize promptly by listening, discouraging acting-out ("temper tantrum") behavior by ignoring it and setting limits on violent behavior. Notice that eventually the child's emotion will be linked to the prompt expression of his spoken word.

At this early age, conditioning most likely results in sustained behaviors that become deeply entrenched in the psyche. Understanding the implications of the gene-environment interaction further supports this hypothesis. Some and probably many developmental and behavioral changes are time dependent — they occur in a certain order and at certain time of life.[2] The expression "missed opportunities" takes on special meaning, if this hypothesis is substantiated.

If behaviors are healthy, such as verbalizing emotions promptly and limiting violent acts, the individual and societal consequences will be profoundly positive. Notice that these childhood experiences are a practice in conditioning. How wonderful it would be if we didn't have to first learn these techniques as adults!

86

Listening Just as Dr. Randolph taught doctors the importance of listening, Alan teaches parents the importance of listening. By example, parents can teach children to listen.

♫♫♫♫♫

As you continue your journey toward your *Energy – the Essence of Environmental Health*, you will see how emotional releases like mine above are as vital as avoidance of toxins or detoxing pollutants. Reducing internal stress levels makes you less reactive as you increase your Accordion Reserve©.

♫♫♫♫♫

PLAYING YOUR ACCORDION

♫♫♫♫

While deconditioning has helped both Alan and me reach a higher level of our individual Accordion Reserve©, we have used positive conditioning in a way that extends to every chapter that follows.

As for me, conditioning solidifies every step of every procedure, including, as an example, *my "Aura"* (Chapter 10), *"Grounding"* (Chapter 11) and so on up to Chapter 21, with my spiritual growth. Always beginning with PHASE III, I have overcome paralysis, learned to control my short-term memory loss, relearned tennis, and most importantly, learned to prevent, stop or minimize environmentally triggered reactions that used to incapacitate me for extended periods of time.

Although I mix and match the techniques from different chapters – according to the desired healing effect, I almost seem to be conditioned to visualize and feel the movement of playing the accordion.

♫♫♫♫

Active, Balanced and Committed To internalize your conditioning as an adult, make a commitment to practice PHASE III CONDITIONING every day to approach deeper levels of relaxation. With time, your mind and body become conditioned to relax at all times yet be braced for unexpected traumas.

Recall the musical analogy of your LUNGS in your body and the BELLOWS in the Accordion (in Chapter 5). Conditioning and de-conditioning are two phases of your body's tolerance that expand your Accordion Reserve©. Remembering to use these techniques during unavoidable exposures helps you maintain an expanded Accordion, thus minimizing your vulnerability to illness.

Meditation/Relaxation Healing contributes to improved Reserve by first influencing Emotional Fitness. If you are just learning PHASE I, and your Reserve is reduced, you may influence your Emotional Fitness just barely enough to overcome the inertia necessary to expand the bellows. With practice, however, you will discover that you can use your Meditation/Relaxation Healing in a positive way to influence all the energy and environmental factors, thus magnifying its impact on your Accordion Reserve©.

SUMMARY

Learn the similarities and differences among these five expressions – conditioning, Meditation/Relaxation, imagery, task and suggestion. They are interdependent and closely aligned, but feel comfortable with these important differences before you proceed to the next chapters:

* Conditioning refers to the process of learning a new behavior, pattern or thought process – as in establishing a habit. Conditioning permits you to complete a sequence of steps with less effort and in less time. A habit is more effectively established through practice (repetition) and reinforcement (encouragement).
* Relaxation (Meditation) is a habit you can learn through conditioning. Meditation/Relaxation allows for the flow

of creative energy, during which you become focused. In a Meditative/Relaxed State it is much easier to perform any task or additional conditioning procedure you wish to accomplish.

* Imagery is a spontaneous, creative awareness that may present as a visual, auditory, tactile, gustatory or olfactory sensation. Imagery is more likely to occur during a Meditative/Relaxed State. Imagery enables you to accomplish a task, thought or process, which may include separate conditioning.

* Tasks are activities that can benefit from additional conditioning to be successfully completed.

* Suggestion is a specific thought that can be introduced during a Meditative/Relaxed State.

Did you practice relaxation, use imagery and condition yourself to learn these important concepts? If you did, you are well on your way to Meditation/Relaxation Healing!

---

[1] Ridley, M. "What Makes You Who You Are," *Time Magazine*, June 2, 2003, pp. 54-63.
[2] Ridley, M. Ibid.

PART IV

Phase-In from Meditation/Relaxation to Energy Healing

AURAS

10
SEEING IS BELIEVING
- Phase IV -
How to Develop the Technique

Prologue

Having mastered your SHORTCUT to Meditation/Relaxation Healing, you are ready to advance to Energy Healing. The expression "Energy Field" has many different names — "Aura," "Auric Field," "Magnetic Field" to name a few, while in the Christian-Judaic belief system, some use the expression "Shield of God."

Some people see their "Energy (Auric) Field"; others feel it; infants appear to depend on it. Others have to relearn their awareness because they suppressed it as they grew up.

Had James Russell Lowell lived today, we would think he wrote *Aladdin's Lamp* to describe Auric Field Healing. For energy "to ward off the cold," Aladdin used "fire enough in my brain;" for visualization, he continued, "I builded...my beautiful castles in Spain." Plain and simple, once you have mastered your auric and visualization techniques, they can be applied for healing, studying, restoring memory, self-anesthetizing *ad infinitum*. Examples can be found throughout the book in appropriate chapters. Each phase has added a dimension to your personal energy management. Thus far, you have learned breathing plus freedom to explore your senses through Body Awareness and conditioning. Experiencing auras is another powerful tool for energy enhancement.

♫♫♫♫♫

As we began to write this book, I had just learned the techniques Natalie will describe below. Spontaneously, I had seen my aura briefly during the first year,

93

but my ability to replicate that first experience on demand is an extraordinary asset. For me, visualizing
auras represents an affirmation of the tactile sense of
energy I feel while I am in PHASE II and III.

♪♪♪♪♪

In Chapter 8, we introduced the concept of Grounding and
the grounded state. Many people can ground themselves by using the SHORTCUT. For example, Alan, an avid runner, was
able to associate his energy with the feeling after a good run.
After only one lesson of relaxation and visualization he could
ground himself and use his energy for healing. However, the
use of his auras has magnified his abilities regardless of his
state of stress.

Caution about Comparison There is no way or reason
to compare my slow progress in energy work (literally taking
years) and Alan's. Disregarding the fact that I was learning by
trial and error to overcome a serious handicap, I did not begin
with the exercise "energy high" that speeded Alan's progress.
As soon as he learned Body Awareness he could make associations that further enhanced his work on his Aura. If Alan and I
had been learning at the same time, comparing his progress to
mine, I would have been seriously hampered.

♪♪♪♪♪

Do not compare yourself or compete with anyone. Do not
compare your own progress even from one day to the next. Many
factors like air quality change daily so that such comparisons could
result in frustration.

♪♪♪♪♪

A Learned Technique Years ago friends kept trying to
convince me that I was psychic, telling me I had a unique talent. I had two abilities: to see auras (others' and mine) and to
pick up other persons' tensions empathetically. Now, I know

that seeing auras is not a unique talent but a learned technique that can be taught to others.

Back in the '70s I was cautioned not to discuss my technique with members of the medical field or I would lose my credibility in Environmental Health – the subject of my books. I knew that scientific research was needed to validate my experience.

Now at last we have scientific papers reporting research on living energy. When I teach people to see their auras, some report that they've seen their auras all along but didn't know what to call their visions. Others become aware of auras as they meditate. However, it is only recently that I learned a method to teach seeing auras to use them for healing.

Off-Focus Vision In the past, I always explained the need to have your eyes off focus to enable you to see your aura, but I could never explain the way to use that off-focus vision to detect your aura. People could either do it on their own or give up the whole process – especially if they were consumed with doubts. Unfortunately for some, the harder they tried, the more frustrated they became; the resulting tension lowered their reserve so there was very little aura to be seen.

♪♪♪♪

GOALS OF EYE EXERCISES

Coordinate regular, consistent practice with breathing exercises to:

* Enhance health of your eyes.
* Improve your vision.
* Hasten your ability to see auras.
* Increase the healing power of your aura/energy.

♪♪♪♪♪

A Negative Becomes a Positive An injured eye successfully ended my search for a method to teach off-focus vision. To strengthen my eye, augment my energy healing and save my vision, I returned to eye exercises, which I had been neglecting for years. My injury confirmed my belief that something positive always occurs to overcome something negative.

Allergic Eyes In the '70's, my ability to see auras began when an ophthalmologist's assistant taught me exercises to strengthen my very allergic eyes. Even the most conventional allergists or ophthalmologists who steadfastly refuse to accept any concepts of Environmental Medicine (EM) acknowledge that eyes are a main target organ for allergies. Hay fever sufferers frequently have runny, itchy eyes plus eye infections and other eye problems. Dust, smoke and mold can also cause eye problems according to conventional physicians.

♪♪♪♪♪

EM specialists recognize that exposure to tar, insecticides, other chemicals and certain foods causes problems as well — blurred vision, loss of ability to focus eye muscles and difficulty opening eyes without prying them open with fingers. Eye problems can also result from emotional stress, for instance, blocking out traumatic scenes and refusing to admit having seen accidents or disasters.

Knowing that allergies often affect the eyes first, you may use them as a beacon to indicate that something in your environment may be causing an allergic reaction. This may indicate the need for using an air filter, a screen in front of your computer monitor, or other suggestions described in Chapter 16. Later you will see how the following exercises can be combined with other techniques to reduce allergic eye reactions. Even healthy eyes need exercise to keep them balanced. The key to seeing auras is healthy, balanced eyes.

Imaginary Huge Clock Imagine a huge clock immediately in front of you. Look down to the imaginary six o'clock.

* Roll your eyes slowly counterclockwise back to six o'clock, visualizing each number.
* Starting again at six o'clock, reverse the movement, slowly rolling your eyes clockwise.
* Look up as high as your eyes can go to an imaginary eleven o'clock, then down to five o'clock, up to one o'clock, and down to seven o'clock, and so on – 10/4, 2/8, 9/3.
* Practice each of the above 3 times.

SEEING IS BELIEVING: FOCUS ON A TARGET

* Choose a target across the room: a doorknob or any small stationary object.
* Focus your eye on the doorknob for a count of 9, enabling your eyes to adjust to the focus.
* After 9 counts, still maintaining the focus on the doorknob, hold your forefinger in front of your doorknob.
* Look at your finger but focus on the doorknob.
* Move your finger slowly away from your nose until you reach arm's length.
* Each eye will see your finger; thus you will be seeing double: two fingers.
* Move slowly with the goal of maintaining, if possible, an even distance between the two versions of your finger as you reach out to arm's length.
* Bring your finger back to position six inches from your nose.
* Repeat (cycles of 3).
* Practice each day (never more than five minutes at a time).

SEEING IS BELIEVING: FOCUS ON YOUR FINGER

* Looking in a direction so you can't see the doorknob, focus on your forefinger as you hold it six inches in front of your nose.
* Still focusing on your finger, turn so your finger is in line with the target.
* Look at the doorknob but focus on your finger.
* Move your fingers slowly away from your nose until you reach arm's length.
* Each eye will see the doorknob; thus you will be seeing double: two doorknobs.
* Move slowly with the goal of maintaining an even distance between the two versions of the doorknob as you reach out to arm's length.
* Bring your finger back to position, six inches from your nose.
* Repeat (cycles of 3).
* Practice each day (never more than five minutes at a time).

♫♫♫♫♫

Serendipity When I held up my forefinger I saw two doorknobs and realized that as my eyes went off focus I was also seeing the aura around my forefinger. Of course! In retrospect I realized that I had developed my ability with auras by practicing the above exercise. You are ready to continue searching for your aura when you continue to see two doorknobs instead of one as you move your finger steadily back and forth.

♫♫♫♫♫

PROCEDURE

Goal: Activate your aura by stimulating your energy.

* Use your SHORTCUT to enter Your Awakening and heighten your ability to function.

* Gently tap your arms, legs, head and chest with your fingers to energize your nerve endings.
* Briskly rub your hands together in a circular motion with your palms touching each other.
* As soon as you have any sensation from the friction, continue the circular motion with your palms still facing each other but gradually moving your hands apart.
* Continue the motion, moving the distances closer, then farther and so on, playing with the sensation.
* Have fun with the variation of the sensation, which in reality is your auric field.

AWAKENING Now you are ready to practice the eye exercise movement using your forefinger to see your aura. Notice how your eyes are off-focus as you see two doorknobs. With your eyes still off-focus on your finger, concentrate on the outline of your forefinger. Even if you see something as vague as the fuzz on a peach, you are seeing your aura.

Comment Many people feel the auric sensation before they can see it. "Philip" was initially frustrated because he could feel his aura so strongly but couldn't see it. I described to Philip how Alan once described his aura with his eyes closed. I could see the same colors in Alan's aura as he described it to me. Philip tried the same technique, and it worked.

Some people say that the human aura looks like the ring of light around the moon; others identify the aura with paintings of the halo. Making a connection to observed phenomena like these can help you, if you have felt frustrated.

Another way of training yourself to see auras, once you have learned to let your eyes go out of focus, is to look at the top of the trees in the distance with your back to the sun. You will probably be able to see the energy or aura of the trees, which will look like a lighter area against the sky, with fluctuations and/or pulsations in the field.

NOW YOU'RE ON YOUR OWN!

We can't tell you what your aura looks like or feels like or how you can use it for healing. Your aura and Your Awakening are as unique as your fingerprints, your DNA and your persona. In fact, your aura changes in color and intensity, depending on your energy, your thoughts and your grounding. However, it may be helpful for you to read how we (Alan and I) and some patients and students see, feel and use auras and Awakenings.

♫♫♫♫♫

<u>Be Creative</u> Let me digress to say that my visualizations and symbols change frequently. Some of the most effective symbols I use are those I've learned from Alan and from very creative patients. Some images come from a past experience, a movie, a poem, a song or something that happens in my daily routine. As you advance, you'll have a sudden inspiration that will be useful to you. Until then, use some of our guidelines.

PLAYING WITH YOUR AURA©

Since I began to experiment with my aura, I have been having fun playing with the variations of it. However, the significance is the immediate response, the increase in my energy and the more effective ability of Auric Healing and helping others to learn to do the same.

As soon as I hold up my hands and spread my fingers, I instantly feel a surge of energy as I watch my aura increase. I hold up my hands, palms facing me, with my fingers spread apart, close but not touching each other. Keeping them aligned, I move my hands away from each other and mimic playing the accordion as I practice my relaxation.

It is interesting to observe the variations of color, intensity and sensations as I change motion and direction. One constant remains. The spaces between the fingers in each hand have a dimmer aura than the space between the aligned fingers (pinky to pinky, forefinger to forefinger). The contrast reminds me of the strings on an old-fashioned corset. You may ask how I know I'm not picking up the colors of objects in the background. Although there's a variety of colors in movement, the pattern between the fingers usually remains constant whether I have a blank white wall in the background or a painting of many colors.

By visualizing a stronger, more vibrant, more colorful aura, I see my aura increasing and mimicking my visualization. I can't explain the phenomenon; I'll leave that to Alan and other scientists. I just enjoy the increased healing power of my aura.

Effective Visualizations Nancy increased her aura by visualizing the scene in the movie "ET" in which ET's "light-streaming" finger healed Elliot's bleeding finger.

Gladys had success visualizing the fading white cloud surrounding the character in the movie "Ghost" as he disappeared into space.

When you practice developing your aura, you feel high energy and also a peaceful relaxation. Is a relaxed energy an oxymoron? Not at all. It is a quiet and peaceful "grounded" vibrational energy flowing from the ground through the soles of your feet, through the top of your head, and beyond, then re-turning along the same path.

This energy extends to every cell in your body, a sensa-tion that makes your body a musical instrument – the Accor-dion. And, of course, you have organs such as the cilia in your ear and your vocal cords which also vibrate. You will soon discover vibrational energy is also healing energy because it balances the parasympathetic with the sympathetic.

♪♪♪♪

Next see PHASE V – "Grounding Your Energy."

11

GROUNDING YOUR ENERGY
- Phase V -
Musical Whispers / Vibrational Overtures

Prologue

To grasp the concept of "grounding your energy," first think of your body as a veritable versatile vibrator, producing music —

* Your cilia (hairs) in your ears, nose, trachea, soft tissues of your oral cavity and throat all vibrate in response to movement of air.
* Your heart beats, pumping blood.
* Your gastrointestinal tract and its sphincters contract, generating movement and passing gas.
* Your bones, blood and body fluids all transmit or generate vibrations.
* Your lungs move air, and your vocal cords vibrate in concert as the air passes over them, producing music.

You can associate each example above, and many others, with one or more musical instruments. Alan identified the Accordion in the last example:

♫♫♫♫♫

Your lungs are the Accordion bellows, and your vocal cords are its reeds.

♫♫♫♫♫

How Alan used his insight of the Accordion is an example of how you can use your insights to promote your own personal healing. Alan's heightened feelings evolved into the powerful message of our musical theme. In Chapter 3, you recall, he recounted how his meditative insight of the Accordion has had such a profound influence on his own personal health. After his initial insight, we regularly meditated and grounded ourselves at the start of each brainstorming session for this book. Alan sometimes spontaneously visualized his grandfather energetically playing the accordion.

The essence of your unique musical body is more eloquent than any manufactured musical instrument, when you learn to ground your energy. Although you were given this gift of energy at the moment of your conception, sensing this energy flow is difficult for some people. Over your lifetime, your body remains aware of this energy, but your conscious mind may need to be reawakened.

When patients are having trouble sensing their energy, Natalie sometimes shows them how they can feel and eventually see energy in all of nature's creatures. The procedures in this chapter will help your body raise its energy to your conscious mind – your own **Awakening**.

Grounding for Environmental Health Bear with us whether you are an expert or novice in grounding techniques. To enjoy Environmental Health (EH), two necessary conditions must occur:

1) You must assess and treat both Environmental and Energy Factors.

2) Then, with practice, using your **SHORTCUT**, your grounding can balance your autonomic nervous system (ANS). Your parasympathetic nervous system and sympathetic nervous system respond appropriately to stimuli and to each other when they are in balance.

A balanced ANS improves your EH.

Need for Grounding Grounding is effective for protection against negatives (others' tensions, environmental exposures and your own negative thoughts). It is even more essential for **Auric/Energy Healing**.

Note of Caution Your energy flow is just like a magnet. It is as unique as your DNA and fingerprints. In an ungrounded state, application of energy-generating treatments may have an undesired effect on your **Accordion Reserve©**. Before experimenting with any energy-generating treatment, be sure you have mastered your own unique **Body Awareness** (Chapter 8).

♪♪♪♪

Philip's Case Philip, an electrical engineer, epitomizes the need for grounding. When he first came to me, I reveled at his energy and aura, a sight to behold, a sensation to experience. Unfortunately, his energy was so wildly ungrounded his electromagnetic sensitivity manifested itself in panic attacks and other serious reactions. He not only gave me permission to use his story, he even encouraged me to describe the progress he has made as an example of damage ungrounded energy can cause.

♪♪♪♪

SCIENTIFIC BACKGROUND

As we write this chapter, articles and books appear almost daily devoted to prayer, spirit and healing. However, it is not always easy scientifically to evaluate the extent to which these virtues contribute to an individual's health, but does it really matter? As written by Dale Matthews, M.D., author of *The Faith Factor,*[1] faith, healing, singing and prayer go hand in hand.

SCIENTIFIC REVIEW

Research identifies positive changes in SPECT scan images of the brain when clergy pray.[2] Schwartz and Russek at the University of Arizona discuss the complex interaction of systems, which is similar to the model we have proposed.[3]

At the same institution, in an article published in the *Archives of Internal Medicine,* Caspi *et al.*[4] suggested that it is time to bridge the gap between those who accept alternative approaches and those who do not. They likened the lack of communication to the Tower of Babel. In this book, we pose many questions to open the dialogue.

Richard Gerber, M.D.,[5] author of *Vibrational Medicine*, extensively researched "esoteric literature" and provided citations that support the functioning systems of meridians and chakras in the human body. Gerber's basic premise is that a living being maintains itself by generating energy and integrates itself with its surroundings by transmitting and receiving energy. In conjunction with the central and peripheral nervous systems, meridians and chakras[6] (see below) function as energy ports in the body, modulating "octaves" of energy so that they can be sensed. (In very simple terms, energy is organized like a musical instrument. Each "C" note is a multiple frequency of itself, i.e. 128 Hertz, 256, 512, etc. These are octaves.)

To give yourself a sense of your own vibrational energy, you can place your fingers in your ears, close your mouth and hum. Not all energy can be heard or seen. Some persons have the unique ability to perceive and transmit energy outside the usual visual and aural (heard) frequencies. When shown your potential to experience other energy, you will improve your sensitivity and awareness.

<u>Meridians</u> Meridians have been shown to function as energy conduits, forming the basis of how acupuncture works to treat many conditions. In fact, one set of meridians runs in the space between blood vessels and the linings of cells. Dr. Rea and Dr. Heine call this area the Ground Regulation System (GRS).[7] When healthy, this complex microenvironment sends energy information at nearly the speed of light. Interacting in this space are many cells and chemical messengers they produce. If the GRS gets congested, energy transmission is interrupted. Eventually, this energy dysfunction results in illness.

In *Vibrational Medicine*, Dr. Gerber further discusses the relationship between "meridians" and "chakras." Using their meridians and chakras, some individuals can sense unseen and unheard energy. While clairvoyants, healers and others are truly gifted in their abilities to sense energy, the rest of us must be re-introduced to skills we probably possessed as infants. We probably relinquished these skills so that we could see and hear the world "out there" more precisely.

Chakras There are seven basic chakras and many more secondary chakras. The lower three are ROOT, SACRAL and SOLAR PLEXUS Chakras, which represent and work on more "down to earth" physical energy. The top three – THROAT, THIRD EYE (Brow) and CROWN Chakras – take on the higher mental energies. The fourth, HEART Chakra, is transitional and represents both physical and mental energies as well as love.

THE UNIVERSAL MODEL OF THE ACCORDION

Recall the Accordion Reserve©. (See **Figures 5-1, 5-2** and **5-3** in Chapter 5.) One handle is influenced by the Environment. The Environment represents the three physical chakras: ROOT (Earth), SACRAL (Water) and SOLAR PLEXUS (Fire). The other handle is Energy. Energy represents the three mental chakras: THROAT, THIRD EYE (Brow) and CROWN. The Bellows represents the remaining chakra – HEART. Symbolically, the HEART Chakra has both physical and mental properties: nurturance by pumping blood to body tissues and by breast feeding, immune function and spirituality as in the emotion of love.

Shakespeare Revisited Could Shakespeare have foreseen the connection of the Accordion Reserve© and the HEART Chakra? Shakespeare's opening line of *Twelfth Night*, "If music be the food of love," expresses our concept of the HEART Chakra; when well-grounded, it opens you to love: love of music, love of art, love of family, love of earth, love of self and love of the Guiding Force.

Additionally, the Heart is physically linked to the Lungs, which are, in effect, a Bellows. When both the Heart and Lungs work efficiently, we feel healthy. The expanded Accordion Reserve©, then, represents the sensation of well-being.

107

Grounding Allows You to Perceive Your Chakras The technique of grounding re-awakens your ability to perceive and sense energy. In the real world, you rely on your usual senses to interact. It is when you also focus on relaxation by grounding that you are able to sense other energies about you.

Whose Tension Is It? As discussed earlier, although you may not recognize it, you are always picking up other people's tensions. Even a baby picks up and withdraws from a mother's tension and develops skin inflammation or colic, etc.

♩♩♩♩♩

Awareness of Tension For years I have been teaching patients how to recognize their body's tensions as their own, to distinguish tension they are picking up from others. It is only after learning to use grounding <u>and</u> auras that patients tell me how quickly they have become aware of other people's tensions being transferred to them.

Patients say they have always been aware of being tense in the presence of certain people and of relaxing when those people leave the room. After they learn to ground themselves using their aura during tense moments they can then pinpoint the tension (headache, pain in the throat, shoulder, etc.) and release it by grounding their energy. Some persons have found that by using a strong vocalized exhalation they can release other people's tensions. Otherwise they now recognize which tension is theirs and use meditation and visualization for relief.

The difference is particularly important if the tense individual is one with whom you have daily contact. For example, "Violet" frequently reported having a serious headache whenever her supervisor walked into the room. She said she had assumed her supervisor intimidated her because her headache disappeared as soon as he left. Now that she can ground herself, she says, "I now know the tension headache is one that I am picking up from my boss."

Keep in mind that the same dynamic is taking place with positive energies. Being around outgoing, happy, relaxed people will give you an energy boost.

♫♫♫♫

CAUTION TO DOCTORS, NURSES AND ALL HEALTH CARE PROFESSIONALS

Protect yourself from toxins and negative energy of your patients. You cannot always smell the toxins released in sweat because patients cover their toxic odors with perfumes and deodorants. Once you have learned to ground your energy you can surround yourself with a protective shield (your magnetic field amplified by grounding), and eventually your body will send spurts of energy to your patients without draining your own *Accordion Reserve*©.

Grounding your energy can be most effective when it is preceded by the SHORTCUT. Even after you advance in your ability to ground yourself, the principle of the *Accordion Reserve*© applies. The greater your reserve and the lesser your degree of stress, the more effective your grounding will be. Unfortunately, the opposite is also true.

♫♫♫♫

Repetition to Emphasize a Point As Alan wrote earlier, sometimes he runs 5 miles or more 5 times a week. After only one lesson of relaxation and visualization he was able to associate his energy with the feeling after a good run. As you recall, he named it The Awakening. He could ground himself and use his energy for healing. However, once he learned to see auras, he found he could ground himself in seconds instead of minutes; the use of the aura has magnified his abilities regardless of his state of stress.

Even I, who still become hyperactive when exposed to certain chemicals, can usually ground and relax myself by enlarging my aura and visualizing my symbols.

♪♪♪♪♪

Find Your Own Pace People who have been working with energy, exercise, yoga, T'ai-chi, Chi Gong (Qi Gong), etc. have the ability to progress much faster than those for whom this is an entirely new experience. Don't attempt to compete with others. Your goal is to find your own pace. Don't even compete with yourself. Remember that each time is different because your **Accordion Reserve**© always fluctuates according to your environmental and energy factors.

Balancing Your Chakras There are many different ways of balancing your chakras, enough to fill several volumes. To help you become your own serendipper for balancing your chakras, let us demonstrate how our method is different. It evolved to include the EH concept of the **Accordion Reserve**© and the **Mind/body/soul/spirit** and was then embellished by our creative visualization and that of our patients.

POWER OF VISUALIZATION

As introduced in Chapter 7, visualization for beginners may consist only of imagination (thought without feeling). Be patient. With practice you will begin feeling **Your Awakening** and graduate to a peaceful energy. At its peak, **Your Awakening** energy through your chakras (charging every cell in your body) will be a peaceful, quiet, spiritual and very effective healing tool.

As we cite examples of visualizations patients experienced during grounding lessons, you will see how we wove successes into a modified system of chakra balancing. Use our suggestions as a guide rather than a fixed method. A guide offers you a choice to develop your own set of patterns whereas a method may be restricting. However, the following models may give you some ideas:

Example 1 "Melodie" said that her faith in God helped her ability to see her energy because it is a gift God gave us all at birth. She visualized herself as a tree and her feet as the trunk, taking energy from the earth. Suddenly she perked up and said, "Oh, there's no mystery to visualization. If you really believe that God gave us at birth the power of healing, the power is in the body, not the mind."

Visualization removes the influence of the mind over the actual process, thus allowing your body to take over the Healing.

Resulting Concept To many of you, grounding is a God-given gift (or use the name of your Guiding Force). Poet Joyce Kilmer committed the same thought to rhyme in the poem "Tree" – "...who lifts her leafy arms to pray." Some patients have said that at final stages of grounding, when they lift their arms they feel the energy of heaven and earth flow from their hands above their head to their feet on the ground and from the ground up through their head. Others report they feel they are in the presence of God, as if they were in a house of worship.

♪♪♪♪

Personal Comment During an intake session, I ascertain the spiritual system of the patient. I have found that those who believe in God respond more quickly when they frequently bring God into the procedure. I attribute my own health improvement to my faith in God. I know I'm called a Pollyanna because I believe that something good comes from the worst adversity. I know that God is always sitting on my shoulder taking care of me, that God is within me.

A friend once asked, "Why are you so special that God sits on your shoulder?" My reply to her: "He's on your shoulder, and He will always be there, and in you. You just have to be aware of His Presence." Because I accept and am always aware of His Presence, I feel God's gift of healing is magnified.

Philip also objected to my statement. He said, "I feel that God is not on my shoulder. He is within me and around me and is omnipresent." Of course I agree. The fact is that I am comforted by the knowledge that He watches over me. Perhaps this is what many mean by "their guardian angel."

Philip's comment brings to mind another patient, who quoted from <u>Corinthians, 3:16-17</u>: "Don't you know that you yourselves are God's temple and that God's spirit lives in you?" One important principle learned from people of many different belief systems is that a force greater than ourselves has given us the power of healing. We cannot allow our blown-up self-importance to impede our progress. By thinking negatively or manipulating a procedure, we strive too hard to succeed and impede the process.

When we use the terms "Energy Healing," "Auric Healing," "Spiritual Healing" or "Self-Healing," we are referring to the process of tapping into the healing power of our Creator, or as some of our patients prefer to say, our "Guiding Force."

♪♪♪♪♪

Example 2 "Celia" visualized her feet in rich black soil and the energy flowing upward through her CROWN Chakra.

Resulting Concept The union of Heaven and Mother Earth for Celia, whose spiritual system was formed on the Jungian concept of the "universal unconscious." During a session Celia said, "I do not have to believe in God to experience grounding. I still experience the union of 'Heaven' ('Infinite') and Mother Earth in my own system of beliefs."

("Heaven," "Infinite" and "Mother Earth" are in quotes to suggest that you may replace them with any phrase that's comfortable for you.)

Celia (like many others with her value system) used the term "false ego." Visualization removes the false ego that stresses you with over-blown self-image and a desperate need to succeed and prove something and overcome the fear of death. No matter what your spiritual convictions are, the symbols of visualization have chemically demonstrated the power of self-healing. Many in the medical establishment will want more scientific research.

Example 3 "Robin" said, "I see many faceless figures rapidly multiplying, just standing there in my CROWN Chakra doing nothing. Then I knew they all represented 'me.' The only way I can be thousands at the same time is that each and every one represents blocked cells in my body. I thought to the figures, 'Come on, get off your duff and start moving,' I felt charged up and the block of tension was broken."

Resulting Concept Multiple symbols combine with even greater effect. The patient's description is analogous to Alan's symbol that each cell represents a battery. The batteries come together to create an extraordinary energy, enhancing the Mind/body/soul/spirit of EH.

VISUALIZING A PROTECTIVE SHIELD

♫♫♫♫

Depending upon the patient's insight or imagery during meditation, I encourage him to make use of that visualization as a means of protection. Thus, in some instances a shield evolves from the image of a hoop skirt of energy, a mummy's wrapping, an energy blanket, a spiral of energy, etc. Alan has had a vision of a coil of energy engulfing and encircling the body's exterior like the caduceus, the symbol of medicine. That circle of energy (his aura) gains strength with grounding.[i]

---

[i] As Natalie and I were editing this section, I commented, "when did I say that?" Natalie reminded me that the caduceus image occurred during my initiation to meditation. This further explains my intuitive responses that we all have, when we free ourselves from controlling with our minds. This example further validates the awareness that many individuals share the same thoughts. Now 6 years later, I was reading *The Five Tibetans*, and was telling Natalie that Kilham had written about the caduceus and its symbolization of energy pathways in our body.

My most successful visualization is the use of God's shield. When I used the term "shield" to one patient, "Dorothy," she sought out several references from the Bible. I quote one from the Old Testament from <u>Genesis 15:1</u>: "...and the word of the Lord came to Abram in a vision saying, 'Fear not Abram, I am your shield.'" One of her quotes was from the New Testament in <u>Ephesians 6:16</u>: "In addition to all this take up the shield of faith with which you can distinguish all the flaming arrows of the evil one."

♫♫♫♫

GENERAL INSTRUCTIONS

1)   Use your own value belief system and give it your own name. Move at your own pace as you feel success with partial commitment. Be cognizant that the sum of all parts is greater than the whole. If you have been committed to PHASE I through PHASE IV and/or other energy factors of EH, or if you have experienced other energy builders (T'ai-Chi, acupuncture, yoga, Qi Gong, etc.) you will have greater success in grounding more quickly.

2)   Always think in first person, visualizing each chakra as you balance it, imagining what it feels like. Think with conviction as if you were actually feeling each step. Gradually your conscious mind will catch up with your body's response to your feeling you have had since birth. We shall guide you through the first two lower chakras, the ROOT Chakra and the SACRAL Chakra. Use the same guide through the rest of your chakras.

3)   Use the SHORTCUT: as you advance you may wish to reach your relaxed state with your own system.

4)   Visualize each step, taking enough time for your body to soak up each thought.

5)   Even before you begin to feel anything, your positive thoughts eventually actualize your sensations (Your Awakening).

114

6)   Slowly keep circling your hand around the chakra you are energizing.

PROCEDURE

* Think something like this: "I'm learning to feel my feet in black soil."
* I am getting a jump-start for every cell (battery) in my feet, ankles, calves and thighs or (since you are dealing with your magnetic field) I visualize a very heavy magnet from under my feet attracting the energy from deep rich soil of the earth.
* I feel the charge of every cell in my ROOT Chakra as the energy circles my ROOT Chakra.
* I feel every cell of my ROOT Chakra spilling over into a shield on the outside of my body, protecting me.
* I see and feel the energy field increasing, widening and gaining strength as it moves down to the earth again, energizing my legs and feet.
* I imagine my energy field being recharged in the rich soil of the earth.
* I feel the energy field moving back up the inside of my legs to the inside of my ROOT Chakra, balancing and recharging the ROOT Chakra.

Comment This is a good time to use the power of your hands, circling your ROOT Chakra, bringing in the sound of your ROOT Chakra "uh" and any other sensations that flow into your Awareness.

* I feel the energy flowing out from my ROOT Chakra as I breathe out and feel it returning more energy as I breathe in, filling my ROOT Chakra.
* I am becoming aware of my energy moving up to my SACRAL Chakra, charging every cell as I circle inside my

SACRAL Chakra, balancing with the energy in my ROOT Chakra.

* My energy is spilling over my SACRAL Chakra outside my body as my shield widens, gaining strength, encircling and protecting my body.

* I return to earth for recharges from the energy of the rich soil of the earth.

Follow the same procedure for each of the chakras including the CROWN Chakra.

After you have visualized charging your CROWN Chakra, visualize a cord or a tree or Alan's streetcar connection reaching upward to an infinite power, using the expression that suits you best. Visualize the power of the Feeling as the energy unites Heaven and Earth, and Your Awakening surges through your body from your head to your toes.

Enjoy Savor the feeling. Think, and repeat 3 times: My Mind/body/soul/spirit is absorbing this Awakening, recording this procedure and conditioning my whole being to be able to reproduce this feeling for healing.

Goal: To unify PHASES I through V by introducing musical sounds.

♪♪♪♪

Even the sounds and pitch of the chakras are unique to each individual energy. I can teach you only the sounds of my chakras, which vary somewhat differently from sounds and pitch I was originally taught. Begin with my guideline sounds and your body will find your own if they vary from mine:

* CROWN Chakra = ē as in eat
* BROW Chakra = ī as in eye or ice
* THROAT Chakra = ā as in ate
* HEART Chakra = ä as in hah

* SOLAR PLEXUS Chakra = ō as in open
* SACRAL Chakra = ü as in boom
* ROOT Chakra = ŭ as in up

♪♪♪♪

As you practice using the chakra sounds, you may begin to vibrate, the sensations of which further enhance Your Awakening.

Revisiting the SHORTCUT

* Begin by activating your nerve ends to stimulate your aura.
* With your knees flexed and your feet flat on the ground, slowly take a deep breath as you spread your arms open wide.
* Visualize opening an accordion.
* Slowly breathe out saying or singing the THROAT Chakra sound ā as in ate.
* Let your hands and shoulders drop.
* Relax, yawn and savor the feeling.
* Repeat twice more, setting a pattern of 3 for conditioning.

Comment You have just combined PHASES I-V.

* Practice only 3 deep breaths at a time to avoid hyperventilating.
* Before repeating each set of 3, relax and practice the procedure for developing PSNS Breathing (See Chapter 7).
* Take turns singing the different chakra sounds, raising the pitch of different notes on the scale.
* With a heightened perception of Body Awareness as you ground yourself, you may experience color, sounds, taste, flavor and touch.

Grounding, music and sensitivity experiences follow in PHASE VI – "Playing with Your Aura©." You will soon see that you have only just begun your musical journey.

SUMMARY

As you read the next chapter, notice how you can use your aura as the healing tool that unifies Part III and Part IV. Use your imagination and your creativity to mix, match and embellish what you have learned from the foregoing chapters and all the techniques you have brought with you from past adventures into healing arts.

---

[1] Matthews DA. 1998. *The Faith Factor.* Penguin Books, New York.

[2] Newberg A, Alavi A, Baime M, Pourdehnad M, Santanna J, d'Aquili E. 2001. The measurement of regional cerebral blood flow during the complex cognitive task of meditation: a preliminary SPECT study. *Psychiatry Research* 106:113-22.

[3] Schwartz GE, Russek LG. 1997. Dynamical energy systems and modern physics: fostering the science and spirit of complementary and alternative medicine. *Alternative Therapies in Health & Medicine* 3:46-56.

[4] Caspi O, Bell IR, Rychener D, Gaudet TW, Weil AT. 2000. The Tower of Babel: Communication and Medicine. *Arch Int Med* 160: 3193-5.

[5] Gerber R. 1996. *Vibrational Medicine.* Bear & Company, Santa Fe.

[6] Kilham CS. 1994. *The Five Tibetans.* Healing Arts Press, Rochester, VT.

[7] Heine H. 1991. *Matrix and Matrix Regulation: Basis for a Holistic Theory in Medicine.* A. Pischinger, ed. H. Heine, Eng. Trans. N. Mac Lean, Brussels, Belgium: Haug International in Rea WJ. 1997. *Chemical Sensitivity* Volume 4. Lewis Publishers, Boca Raton, FL.

12
PLAYING WITH YOUR AURA©
- Phase VI -
Your Healing Instrument

Prologue

♫♫♫♫♫

The thrill and rapture of feeling my energy flow and seeing it for the first time was a magical "high." For me, it was every bit as invigorating as a runner's "second wind." Capturing the sensation and applying it to our daily stressful lives is a joy that I will treasure forever. I recall the gossamer wisps of energy shimmering, extending from my fingertips and streaking skyward. As illusory as it seems, the infinite sensation of my arms suspended weightless above my head still tingles my spine whenever I play with my aura.

♫♫♫♫♫

How would you like to experience holding in your hands something that feels like a heavy brick, but looks like a soap bubble? Many of us have similar experiences when we play with our auras. Read on and savor the fascination with your own aura.

PLAYING

♫♫♫♫♫

When we experiment with new methods to use our auras, Alan and I are like big kids who never grew up. We approach Playing with Your Aura© as a flashback to childhood, playing games (not learning techniques). Have fun! As I watch Alan, he's like a little boy playing with a new toy — the excitement, the exuberance, almost child-like glee.

119

Suddenly, his scientific mind takes over; the doctor in him begins to evaluate possible medical applications and physiological implications of what we are doing. Off the top of his head, he cites scientific research we can quote – papers that validate what we are experiencing. Sometimes his agile mind suddenly recognizes a way to modify a mainstream treatment by applying a technique we've discussed in *Energy – the Essence of Environmental Health.*

When I was teaching my niece Trish to find her aura, I described my feeling as a heavy brick. I told her of a patient changing the brick into a stone from a lake and feeling the dripping waters releasing negative ions. Trish looked at her aura, focused on the feeling and visualized a cushion. I took up the challenge immediately and used Trish's cushion as God's shield. It is soft, firm, protective and secure.

The real fun begins as a game when you can share Playing with your Aura© with others.

Reminder As I guide you through the steps that have helped us and some patients to reach the aforementioned powerful healing tool, remember that my basic guide is only a beginning step. Your own creativity, visualization and past experience with visualization and/or energy (T'ai-chi, yoga, Qi Gong, etc.) will lead you to your own individual images. As you proceed you may wish to incorporate some ways we use auras for healing (see later in this chapter).

♪♪♪♪♪

As noted earlier, "seeing is believing." Feeling and sensing are also believing.

Continuity Revisited As a beginner, precede the following instruction by using your SHORTCUT to Your Awakening, practicing seeing your aura and grounding yourself. As previously noted, some patients can sense or feel their aura before seeing it. Paradoxically, after they feel it, they learn to see it.

PROCEDURE

* Gently tap arms, legs, head and chest with fingertips to energize your nerve endings.
* Gently slap your hands together.
* Slowly move your hands and rub them together in a circular motion. Move your hands apart about two inches, palms still facing each other.
* Continuing the circular motion, imagine each hand as a magnet as you slowly pull your hands apart 4 to 6 inches.
* Push your hands together back to 2 inches apart.
* Repeat twice more to maintain the conditioning pattern of 3.
* Focus on the feelings in your hands. You may feel heat, cold, hands being pulled together, hands pushed apart, tingling, etc. or a combination of many sensations.
* At first, you may not be able to distinguish what you are feeling. This lack of sensation may indicate that at this particular time your Accordion Reserve© is very low. Even so, go on to the next step after you have practiced for three minutes.
* Again with your hands 2 inches apart, move your hands in a slightly circular motion with palms facing each other, hands close to your solar plexus (diaphragm) but parallel to the floor.
* Once you feel a strong sensation, move your hands (palms facing each other) back and forth, pushing away and pulling together to activate the magnetic pull or push strengthening the sensation.

SEEING AURAS REVISITED

♪♪♪♪♪

Recall how frustrated Philip was when he could feel but not see his powerful aura until he closed his eyes. Then Philip opened his eyes. This time, he watched his aura grow and observed: "Oh, I've seen this before, but it was so subtle and

without color that I did not associate it with my magnetic field."
As Philip's aura intensified, I could see which of his chakras
were blocked because they lacked color and size. After that he
was able to unblock those chakras and reach his goal of
learning to ground himself.

♪♪♪♪♪

Exception As previously cited, Philip was one of many who
first had to see and feel his aura before he could use it to ground himself. As Philip's confidence grew, so did his aura, and he rapidly
learned to use his aura for grounding and healing. He has already begun to invent his own method of playing with his aura and increasing
his Accordion Reserve© by reducing reactions in a stressful situation.

♪♪♪♪♪

Once you feel the powerful magnetic sensation in your
hands (what I call my brick), even if you can't yet see it, invent
ways for you to play with it. I begin with the palms of my hands
facing each other about two to four inches apart. Keeping the
same distance, I imagine causing friction as I move both hands
clockwise, palms still facing each other. Gradually, I move my
hands further apart, making my brick larger. Then the fun
begins. I move my brick to the right, to the left, upward,
downward and watch and feel my brick move with my hands.

In fact, you can maximize your energy by adding your
music (chakra sounds) as you play with your aura.[i]

Select a melody and "hum" it, using the sound that
stimulates the chakra representing your symptomatic organs.
In **Table 12-1** below, for example, "o" refers to the small
intestine in the SOLAR PLEXUS Chakra. So use "o" if you are

---

[i] Better yet, sing your chakra sounds while standing ankle-deep in a tub of water.
Or you could do this while taking a shower. This technique increases your
grounding ability because water is a better conductor of vibration and sound than
air.

having a "gas problem." Use "ā" for the THROAT Chakra if you are hoarse. For migraine, try "ē" or "ī."

CHAKRA	VOWEL SOUND
CROWN	ē as in eat
BROW	ī as in eye or ice
THROAT	ā as in ate
HEART	ä as in hah
SOLAR PLEXUS	ō as in open
SACRAL	ü as in boom
ROOT	ŭ as in up

Table 12-1. Chakra sounds. Use sounds to maximize your Energy while playing with your aura.

Now you are ready to sequence all SIX PHASES into one procedure. With your musical input, your functioning energy generator will transform into an energy healer.[i] In Chapter 21, you will explore adding spirituality to this powerful instrument.

Color - My New Toy For years the colors of my aura were almost imperceptible. Then, one night before retiring, to clear a nasal condition, I combined visualization with a long hot shower — water jetting full force on the top of my head. I followed the shower with meditation and playing with my aura.

---

[i] You can transfer healing bioenergy from your moving hands to other parts of your body. This process is probably a form of electromagnetic induction, analogous to the way an electric generator works. In an electric generator, mechanical force sets a magnet and its magnetic field in motion (analogous to your moving, bioenergetic hands). In turn, this moving magnetic field induces an electric current (electrical energy) in a nearby coiled wire (analogous to a nearby body part). This energy transfer occurs across empty space; the magnet and coil do not touch each other. This process is analogous to your moving hands inducing healing energy in a nearby body part.

123

That night as I held my hands palms facing me, digits spread apart but pointing at each other, pinky to pinky, etc., I began playing with my aura. Stretched like steamy ribbons from matching paired fingers, the colors formed an arch, mimicking a rainbow. My rainbows had the vagueness of pastels, hues gently streaming towards each other – distinct, yet muted. Soon after my aura colors became clearly defined.

Have fun! Try it yourself.
♫♫♫♫

Comment At this point, it is still not necessary to see your aura, in order to sense it, but with practice, you can do what Philip did. While some people readily detect their chakra colors, the color links are not always identical. See **Table 12-2** below for an example of colors for chakra healing.

CHAKRA	COLOR
CROWN	Violet
BROW	Indigo
THROAT	Blue
HEART	Green
SOLAR PLEXUS	Yellow
SACRAL	Orange
ROOT	Red

Table 12-2. **Chakra colors. Colors can be used for healing. (Adapted from Gerber R., 1996, *Vibrational Medicine*, p. 275.) Visualizing color can help maximize your energy while playing with your aura.**

♫♫♫♫♫

As we edited this book we continued to discover new creative insights. As I sat in a swivel desk chair, playing with my aura, I aligned my fingertips. Then, I started spinning myself slowly. Wonderfully, beautifully and most energetically, streams of color passed between my fingers. Were my eyes deceiving me? Again I replicated the sensation, as I rotated in the opposite direction and came to a halt. And then I gave voice to my amazement: "Just like a kid." Of course, Natalie gave it a try. She too was fascinated by how powerful and colorful her aura had become. I was able to detect her aura much more readily after she had spun herself.

Try this swivel maneuver to enhance your aura.
♫♫♫♫♫

Your Healing Tool - Visualizations Revisited First review the visualization suggestions and techniques described in Chapters 9, 10 and 11. Combine those techniques and those of your own creation by adding the power of your aura with your chakra sounds.

Power of Your Aura It is believed that your aura is the visual image of your energy. Machines (automobiles, computers, your body, etc.) function at maximum capacity in direct connection with their level of energy. Clinically we find that playing with your aura and grounding with your aura increase and stabilize your energy.

♫♫♫♫

Your Aura for Prevention (Natalie's Nuggets for Prevention) Many patients felt lost when our allergist, Dr. Eloise Kailin, moved away from suburban Washington, D.C. We learned the validity of the maxim "Necessity is the mother of invention," improvising, using grandmas' remedies and sharing successes with others.

Although I still apply many of the early substitutes, I find them more powerful now that I add my aura energy. My recovery has speeded up since I began using my aura to maximize every function of my energy. Take what you like from what follows. Improve by making changes and additions to suit you.

  * Food, Supplements and Water – Whenever possible I play with my aura as I eat, drink or swallow supplements. Only

lasting a matter of seconds, my aura play increases my ability to digest food because I'm eating in a relaxed state.

* Several times a week I indulge myself! I briefly play with my aura as I pick up an apple, feeling energy from its color, texture and aroma. As I nibble on the apple, I visualize its energy, delight in its crunching rhythm and thank God for my food. I revel in my increased energy and find strength in my aura. I do the same with supplements, especially my Vitamin C.

* I also practice relaxation techniques and Playing with my Aura© whenever possible while:
    * Doing chores (dishes, laundry, tidying the house, etc.)
    * Showering (especially during a bath)
    * Watching TV
    * Waiting at a red light while in the car
    * Walking and exercising
    ♫♫♫♫

<u>*Your Aura for Treatment*</u> First, here is an example of ways you can build on others' symbols and visualization.

♫♫♫♫

I demonstrated to Alan how I visualize a white light entering through my CROWN Chakra. If I sense that I am experiencing negative thoughts, emotions or a toxic overload, I imagine securing them in balloons. Next I visualize the white light expelling the balloons from the involved chakra and destroying the spheres. I then visualize sealing the chakra so that the stressor will not return.

The next day, as Alan was running five miles, he visualized not balloons but bubbles (like effervescent bubbles of Randolph's bi-salts and Rea's tri-salts, which are the Environmental Medicine substitutes for Alka Seltzer Gold™) and seeing toxins flow out in beads of perspiration.

Since then I have used Alan's bubble symbol as a shield before I break my diet when eating out, before I enter a polluted area, or before I work with a toxic overloaded patient. Moreover, the bubble symbol is a very important aid in treating reactions.

Caution Lest you become discouraged when your methods fail or are less powerful at times, remember that success depends on the level of your Accordion Reserve©.

When my Accordion Reserve© is full, I prevent, minimize and overcome serious reactions more quickly than I overcome a minor reaction when my Accordion Reserve© is low. Reminder: visualization is most effective when you are relaxed and your energy is grounded. It is also worth repeating that visualization keeps you focused on symbols and dissuades you from "trying too hard."

To help yourself through a crisis of craving a "forbidden" food LISTEN to YOUR BODY and practice Auric Healing.

Auric Healing for Insect Bites For a high histamine reaction (especially insect bites and pollen):

I experienced two episodes during which I was attacked by a swarm of mosquitoes (one in Mexico after an earthquake and one in Florida on a golf course). In each instance, I used a hat to beat off the mosquitoes; both times my white hat turned bloody red (my blood from the mosquitoes I killed!).

In another instance, one bite on my face made me swell to elephantine proportions. Unable to use antihistamines, I had to find a way to protect myself. I was put to the test halfway home from a tennis court where I had been bitten in the eye. As I pulled off the road my face swelled so rapidly and painfully that I wondered how I'd get home.

To avoid panic I began to meditate and ask my body for a symbol to use for antihistamines. Spontaneously I thought of a commercial about Benadryl™ acting as a histamine blocker. I began to visualize blocking the histamines.

* As I played with my aura, I pictured myself running down my high school corridor. Along the way I was vehemently slamming all the locker doors. I visualized the locker doors trapping the histamines.
* For histamine already released, I visualized drinking bi-salts. I pictured Alan's bubbles coming out of my eyes, nose and skin.
* As my aura began to look like steam pouring out of my fingertips, I visualized the steam penetrating and neutralizing the histamines.
* I have no idea how long it took, but I could finally drive home. After meditating several times during the day, the next day my face was back to normal. In the past it used to take a week or two for the swelling to recede.

Research Needed I have not had another incident of a swollen face since then. Coincidence? Who knows? As a preventive measure, before leaving the house I meditate briefly and revisit the above sequence. Whenever possible I'm careful to avoid areas infested with mosquitoes. However, I do not allow insects to keep me housebound. This experience is probably another example of "mind over matter." As in our previous citations, is this an instance of experience turning off certain genes?[1]

Reminder Whenever you use any self-healing techniques remember that it is a gift given to you at birth. Otherwise, your false ego will step in, making the procedure less productive because your mind will take over instead of your body.

I must digress to demonstrate how other modalities that follow similar procedures have a common thread. Case in point is a patient for whom chakras were at first so foreign that she needed extra motivation. One day, very excited, she brought me a *Time Magazine* article[2] about yoga to show me an illustration that compared Eastern View Chakras and Meridians with Western View Nervous System and Glands, showing the correlation with the organs and the glands.

What caught my eye was the statement that, especially in the first yoga sessions, students may have trouble suppressing those competitive ways – and force themselves into a gym rat race. With yoga, T'ai-Chi, Chi Gong (Qi Gong), as with our program, competition is not only contraindicated, it can be destructive. Competition implies that you must be best, you must be perfect, and to be these, you must try harder. That is why I tell patients, "Forget 'try'." Instead, practice. And a better way to practice is to give the power of success to your Guiding Force. That removes your ego in the same way visualization keeps your focus off trying.

PROCEDURE: GROUNDING WITH YOUR AURA

* Once you can feel the heavy pull of your magnetic field, you can add the weight to your grounding, using a little imagination.
* Imagine pulling heavy magnets out of the ground under your feet.
* Pull the magnets up by using the image of your energy ball weight (what I now call "God's Shield").
* Place your hands, palms up on each side of your body, beginning with your feet, up along your legs.
* Stop briefly at each chakra.
* Visualize your energy ball weight circling each chakra.
* Once you reach your CROWN Chakra, push your hands up above your head as if lifting weights, as if reaching the "North Pole" of your magnet.
* Reverse the order, pulling your magnets to the earth under your feet (South Pole of your magnet).

NATALIE'S TRAUMATIC CHALLENGE

♪♪♪♪♪

While working on this chapter, my mental attitude, "turning negative into positives," was put to a test. I experienced a dramatic challenge that tested my belief that every adversity, no matter how traumatic the experience, is beneficial. In "My Story," Chapter 2, you read some of the obstacles I have had to overcome. (What I wrote is just the tip of the iceberg that other early "canaries" and I had to overcome by trial and error.)

Picture this scenario — I'm enjoying my house, my diet, my social life, my work and having a ball working with my co-author on this book. The future looks even brighter.

SLAM! BANG!

Decline in health, gradual deterioration, sluggishness, diet, erratic sleep habits, but I can't find a pattern. Rash begins slowly, blossoming out in small areas. Rash spreads all over except my face. Rash itches - burns - aches - worse when I shower and when I eat. Awaken several times at night – I'm scratching myself. Can't stand smell of freshly washed clothes. Suspect my water filters must have overloaded. Condition becomes critical. Have to fight negative thoughts.

First Corrective Steps Increase nutrients. More time meditating, but can't exercise. Relief from meditation lasts about 1 and 1/2 hours. Start bathing in bottled spring water. Begin testing everything I eat, touch, smell – no pattern. Symptoms continue.

Bad News My house is at the end of the pipeline, and dirt cannot be flushed out via the nearest fire hydrant. Washington Suburban Sanitary Commission (WSSC) can't or won't help. WSSC says my water is up to standards! Yet the water quality disrupted my entire filter system, including the whole-house filter and the additional filters in my kitchen and showers. Black chips of filter residue come through my faucet.

The Cause Discover water main break very close to my house. Even my filtered water smells of chlorine. Have to change filter again in three weeks.

Corrective Step Change water filter replacements.

Deteriorating Health Complications Can't do detox bath — confined to using bottled water for bathing and washing vegetables. Sleep deprived. React to food in freezer — foods previously washed in the contaminated filtered water. React to chlorine in the air even though I've purchased an extra air filter. React to clothes recently washed in machine. Tests show a bacteria (Pseudomonas *aeruginosa*) is growing in my GI tract.

TURNING NEGATIVES INTO POSITIVES

The Challenge As you can see from **Table 12-3** (see later), I had to turn negatives into positives. You will note that in the right column of the table I limited the scope of my symptoms, rather than expanding them through fear. Then I focused on My PROGRESS, My Energy/Spiritual Healing, and my ability to recover. I recognized that this apparent setback was another challenge. It was an opportunity to test my energy work in a crisis situation.

I noticed that even my dreams took a positive turn. Instead of waking from my recurring dream that I was clawing my skin, I dreamed I was playing with my aura using my vagus nerve.[i] That image had its roots in our earlier discussions (see Chapter 6) about the effects of the vagus nerve on the autonomic nervous system (a vehicle of our energy work).

---

[i] The 10th Cranial nerve, which sends parasympathetic nervous system messages to most organs.

	NEGATIVE THOUGHTS	POSITIVE THOUGHTS
My Skin Reactions	If my outer skin is erupting, what havoc is inside?	Thank God, my face is unaffected.
My Symptoms of Chemical Sensitivity	My itching is causing me more distress than my paralysis and my dysphagia caused me when my illness began.	My Spiritual Healing is giving me progressively longer periods free of itching.
My Environment	The house is ruined. I have nowhere to go.	I built my oasis once. I can do it again.
My Outlook on Life	I'm in a no-win situation. My fears for the worst outcomes have returned.	Environmental Medicine (EM) has advanced since 1966. I can access many EM doctors, including Alan.

Table 12-3.   Emotions run deep and strong. Turning negatives into positives.

Did I experience immediate success? No. At first, in my desperation and fear, I was <u>trying</u> – my mind and my false ego were going to prove something. When I recognized that <u>trying</u> was interfering with my healing, I changed my approach, began breathing with the SHORTCUT and played with my aura. Like a stream of consciousness, images flashed into my mind, one at a time. My visualization pattern kept changing:

My body was the accordion.
* The handles were the North Pole and the South Pole magnets.
* *Pushing and pulling, the magnets opened and closed my body.*

* *The vagus nerve became the accordion.*

I visualized the vagus nerve as an Accordion/Aura moving through my chakras. As I drifted off to sleep, my last recollection was that my fingers and toes shed the painful cold, even as my body and arms relinquished their intense burning heat at the sites where I felt itching moments before.

Did my problem disappear over night? No! The contaminants were still in my house. But I did sleep through the night for the first time. Alan and I are convinced that the procedure did help restore my Accordion Reserve© to some extent, although research is needed to explore that. Be that as it may, I did get relief and continue to do so even though, as I write this, the water pollution still exists.

BENEFITS RESULTING FROM A TRAUMA

* I replaced my defective water filtration system with one more capable of filtering the unsatisfactory water in my area.
* I found a more effective healing/grounding procedure for me and perhaps for others.
* Since the vagus nerve and the parasympathetic nervous system have effects on the eye, I will use this visualization to help me heal my eye, previously injured by blunt trauma from a tennis ball. Perhaps with this experience, we can encourage in-depth research on the effect of visualization and the Accordion Reserve©.
* The experience gave us a vehicle to demonstrate the efficacy and powerful concept of the Accordion Reserve©.

TAPPING INTO PATIENTS' CREATIVITY

My healing ability has reached new heights as I fine-tune my procedure (Parts III and IV) by modifying and embellishing creative ideas from patients, students and, of course, Alan. To help you do the same, I have asked for and been granted permission to demonstrate how you can do the same.

Automatic Pilot "Jennie" finally learned how to reduce and sometimes stop emotional reactions caused by chemicals, molds and foods. As she searched for a way to bring fast relief, she suddenly used the term Automatic Pilot. Many other patients independently used the same term.

How I Personalized Automatic Pilot Every year I visit my brother Ellery and his wife Lila in Minnesota, where pollution is much less. On a windy day, I sat on the dock taking in the negative ions of pristine lake water. Over the reverberation of rolling waves against a barrier of rocks and the beach, I grounded myself and played with my aura. As I recorded meditation tapes for conditioning, healing and sleeping, I programmed myself to initiate instant grounding and relive the setting just by thinking Automatic Pilot. I frequently play the tape in bed before going to sleep because I believe those who say that the brain learns messages even while we sleep. I conditioned myself to learn from the tape even after I fall asleep.

Several times a day before eating, driving a car or any tense moment, I take three relaxation breaths, think Automatic Pilot, and immediately I am grounded. (More about automatic grounding later.)

Audio/Visual Reinforcement In the stifling summer heat, pollution and high humidity ("Dog Days of August") I frequently need a "refresher course." As I listen to my lakeside meditation tape, I can reproduce and augment the peaceful beauty, the cool pleasant breezes by looking at snapshots of the lake, beach and woods at the site around my vacation hideaway.

Use your audio/visual refreshing experiences to reproduce and/or heighten Your Awakening.

THE NETI POT [i]

Philip introduced me to the ceramic Neti Pot (shaped like Aladdin's lamp), which is much more efficient than the system I had always recommended for additive-free salt water nasal cleansing.

Philip told me the Neti Pot has given him great relief during the pollen season. It is effective for dust, mold, and other mucus-causing problems.

My Variation After successfully using the instructions that came with the Neti Pot, I experimented, adding my own embellishments:

* Before using the Neti Pot, I invoke Automatic Pilot.
* After following the manufacturer's instructions, I take a few sips of hot water, clearing my throat after each sip.
* As I prepare my breakfast and nutrients, I slowly drink two eight-ounce glasses of hot water, clearing my throat and nose from residue stimulated by hot water.

Results My hearing, vision and digestive tract have gradually improved. Automatic Pilot is just one term or symbol to elicit immediate grounding (your best Awakening). Try the term and then see if you have a better symbol.

Unless my Accordion Reserve© is extremely deflated, Automatic Pilot conditions me so that I immediately feel my mind and ego turning control over to my body and the "Powers That Be." More about Automatic Pilot in later chapters.

---

[i] Himalayan Institute (1-800-832-4547) has excellent instructions and pictures. Many other companies also carry the Neti Pot.

SUMMARY — EVER -CHANGING

My aura, Body Awareness symbols, visualizations and procedure variations – everything is in a constant flux. My aura always responds to whatever visualization or insight I have at the moment. My healing always responds to my aura. With practice you can reach the same contact with your visualization or whatever you call your trigger. (Also see Chapter 21 for my spiritual trigger).

♫♫♫♫♫

Natalie relies on Playing with Your Aura© much more than I. She is more conditioned to using it than I am.

When I am aware of stress I:

* Begin my position and breathing exercises – yoga-like relaxation – enhancing the responses of the parasympathetic and sympathetic nervous systems.
* Visualize fizzy bubbles (like "tri-salts") – releasing my stress.
* Visualize the handles of the Accordion (representing the stressors).
* Defuse the intensity of stress by playing the accordion with my hands.
* Sense energy surging between my hands.
* Feel my arms - floating and weightless.
* See sequential colors with my eyes closed -
  * Usually a full green field - for healing.
  * Pinpoint red for CROWN Chakra energy, which generates an entire body flow of energy, when I feel a tingling flush.
  * Pinpoint purple - for insight.
* Vocalize - sometimes a cry, which opens my THROAT Chakra.

An example of this pattern occurred when I developed "writer's block" while editing Chapter 3: "My Story." That stress resulted in the above healing sequence and helped me understand why I had the block. Of course, the edits flowed smoothly after I "Played with My Aura."

You should also know that an example such as mine is not always immediate in its onset, nor is its healing 100%. I needed two images before I could see my aura in this example. My next stress relief experience may be identical, faster, slower or have a different set of images. Notice also that the colors I relate to my chakras differ from those in **Table 12-2** above.

With your conditioning process, practice improves healing. Expect that your conditioning process will frequently change, as you trust yourself to relax and release your ego. Keep a fresh perspective and allow your images to flow freely, like a sparkling mountain stream. Your Auric Healing is a spontaneous and creative moment. Your power comes from your Mind/body/soul/spirit through your Guiding Force.

♫♫♫♫♫

---

[1] Ridley, M. "What Makes Us So Special?" *Time Magazine,* June 2, 2003.
[2] Corliss, R. "The Power of Yoga," *Time Magazine,* April 23, 2001.

PART V

The Beginning of Harmony

ENERGY RESOURCES

13
SLEEP
- Meditation -
Prescription for Healing Sleep

Prologue

♫♫♫♫♫

"Rise and Shine!" The trumpets sounded "Reveille." That is how I remember waking up at camp. We slept on an open-air platform tent – chilly but invigorating. I was excited to start the new day. Fond memories positively influence my ability to sleep even now. Our most important life function, sleep, allows for daily rejuvenation, healing and growing. In other words, optimal sleep expands your Accordion Reserve©.

♫♫♫♫♫

SLEEP - RHYTHMS AND DISTORTIONS

With our sincerest apologies to comedian Jeff Foxworthy, we offer the new expression "Fog Head" (one whose sleeplessness causes "brain fog").

- ⏰ If you sleep during the day and are awake at night, you might be a Fog Head.
- ⏰ If you work at night, and sleep during the day, you might be a Fog Head.
- ⏰ If you sleep at odd times, you might be a Fog Head.
- ⏰ If you sleep in short spurts, you might be a Fog Head.
- ⏰ If you have a chronic illness, you might be a Fog Head.
- ⏰ If you belch and your chest burns in the night, you might be a Fog Head.
- ⏰ If you have muscle or joint pains that scream out in the night, you might be a Fog Head.

- ⏰ If you have a bladder that beckons incessantly at night, you might be a Fog Head.
- ⏰ If your heart pounds in a syncopated rhythm at night, you might be a Fog Head.
- ⏰ If your spouse snores like a freight train, you just might be a Fog Head.
- ⏰ If you feel you are gasping for your last breath in the night, you might be a Fog Head.
- ⏰ If you feel like a raging bull at night, you might be a Fog Head.
- ⏰ If you are saddled with "shift work," you really are a Fog Head.
- ⏰ If you are a tired parent, frequently disturbed by a crying child at night, oh boy, are you a Fog Head!
- ⏰ If you have insomnia, you definitely are a Fog Head!
- ⏰ Get the picture!!!

Because sleep disturbance is such a serious problem, we tried to <u>inject</u> a little humor. This is an important lesson – laughter is still the best medicine – no matter how it is prescribed. Always think of something amusing to turn negatives into positives.

Sleep disturbance is such a pressing predicament because your nervous system has difficulty adjusting to frequent disruptions at night. It is like experiencing continuous jet lag. As you would expect, chronic sleep distortions adversely affect the autonomic nervous system (ANS) and *vice versa,* and result in a shrinking Accordion Reserve©.

However, you have learned the power of conditioning. Now learn how to maintain or correct your sleep habits. Read on!

SLEEP, EXERCISE AND NUTRITION ARE INTERDEPENDENT

<u>*Sleep Influences Exercise*</u> When sleep deprived over a long period, you lack the proper energy for healthy, strenuous exercise. It is possible to perform, but just not as well. It is a universal truth that

142

children who are tired have more accidents and frequently end up at the emergency room.

Sleep Influences Nutrition If too tired, babies will not eat (that applies even more to adults if they have to prepare the food.) Babies who do not eat will not grow. Since growth is the most identifiable characteristic, it is obvious why sleep is so important. Patterns carry into adulthood.

Exercise Influences Sleep Intensity, timing and duration of exercise and nutrient consumption relative to exercise influence sleep patterns. You are unique. Through practice with **Body Awareness**, your body will teach you what it needs.

♫♫♫♫♫

Example In the past my exercise needs were based mostly on "detoxing" – rigorous daily programs of "burning fat" that released toxins, which my liver processed for elimination. In retrospect I compensated by cutting back on sleep. I paid a price by developing musculoskeletal injuries and more severe autonomic neuropathy.

As I have healed my ANS, I observed that my need to exercise vigorously has decreased, while my requirement for continuous sleep has increased. Although my schedule often interferes, I remind myself to follow the principles outlined in this chapter on promoting a positive sleep environment: As I focus with relaxing images like my blue sphere, I fall asleep promptly, and I awake without an alarm, when my body tells me. Most of the time I still have adequate time for my morning exercise routine.

♫♫♫♫♫

Nutrition Influences Sleep In Chapter 14, you will learn about our approach to nutrition, and in Chapter 15, you will appreciate the interaction of exercise and nutrition. Recall from Chapter 5, that the Energy Handle of the Accordion relates sleep, exercise, nutrition and relationships. Not surprisingly, what you eat and when you eat it affects the quality and quantity of sleep. This discussion has the potential to become quite involved depending on individual needs. Two examples will suffice to stimulate further thought.

Example 1 You have a tendency to low blood sugar. Low blood sugar triggers adrenalin to raise blood sugar. Adrenaline is a neurotransmitter for the sympathetic nervous system (SNS). Therefore, low blood sugar during sleep may result in early awakening, sweats, seizures, headaches and profound drowsiness in the morning. An adjustment in food selections might be to include a small protein and fat snack (with or without carbohydrate) before bed. For some people who eat dinner at 6-8 p.m., a prolonged period without food may generate the same outcome as low blood sugar.

This same approach of eating a protein/fat snack before bed can result in the need for less sleep, yet arising more alert.

Example 2 You are sensitive or allergic to several foods or chemicals. During an exposure, you may develop symptoms of SNS overactivity. As in the example above, sleep interruptions are likely to occur.

CONDITIONED SLEEP PATTERNS BEGIN IN INFANCY

♫♫♫♫♫

Sleep habits are acquired during the earliest days of infancy. Newborns may sleep 16 or more hours a day. Parental attitudes about sleep influence infant sleep patterns. While some experts may disagree, I encourage parents to set a goal of "8 hours at 8 weeks." In other words, an otherwise healthy, full-sized 2-month-old should be able to sleep 8 <u>consecutive</u> hours without awakening and requiring nutrition. This goal often is accomplished by chance, but a conditioning program often yields the results.

Why is this a desirable goal? In my opinion, this routine forms a stable sleep foundation for infancy, childhood and beyond. If you already have such a base, then you can always rely on it, should you experience a <u>temporary</u> (think positively!) interruption in quality sleep.

In the newborn period, babies will most often wake to feed every 2 to 4 hours. However, with a very filling "meal" some babies will tend to sleep longer. If that happens during daytime hours (when you are awake), then to that baby it "feels like night." Wouldn't it be desirable to encourage that longer sleep interval to occur at the time when you yourself are trying to sleep? That's where your active participation in conditioning pays off.

The principles are similar to those you learned about potty training and the "terrible two's" in Chapter 9: "Conditioning."

1) When your baby wakes during daytime, pay attention by responding promptly to fussy crying that seems to be hunger-triggered. Feed promptly. Talk, play, sing and engage the baby by changing his diaper, picking him up and so on. Continue attention activity after the feeding is complete. This liveliness positively reinforces "awake."

2) Make a distinction between daytime awake and nighttime sleep by "selectively ignoring" the baby at night. I don't really mean "ignore." Instead reduce attention to the minimum necessary to accomplish the "business" of feeding without all the fanfare. In other words, when baby awakes at night, respond to <u>vigorous</u> crying only when baby really <u>wants</u> to be fed. Minimize verbal cues for attention and playing. Minimize handling such as changing diapers unless necessary. Discourage attention after the feeding is complete. Return the baby to his sleep environment before he falls asleep during feeding.

3) The contrast between attention and relative "non-attention" becomes conditioned – attention equals daytime awake and non-attention equals nighttime sleep.
♫♫♫♫

WHEN ADULT SLEEP PATTERNS NEED FINE-TUNING

Could it be that you were one of those infants who was not conditioned to sleep successfully in the newborn period? Were you actually conditioned to confuse day and night?

<u>Dealing with Negative Emotions</u> Intuitively, you understand the importance of sleep and the daily consequences of successful as well as unsuccessful sleep. Unfortunately, you may be

so driven to succeed that you introduce failure. Frustration and anger follow, provoking negative thoughts that further interrupt your sleep. If you are caught in this trap, the word "sleep" gains new meaning.

Go no further than the New Testament to appreciate the importance of going to sleep without anger: "Let Not The Sun Go Down on Thy Wrath."[i] Anger, fear, and general negative thoughts are the three emotions that can be blamed for more sleepless nights than all other things combined. As we present our guidelines for dealing with anger, you can adopt ideas for the other causes of sleeplessness. However, don't wait until bedtime, letting anger fester all day long. There are several ways to deal with anger.

Visualizations Revisited A good first step combines grounding with relaxation techniques, meditation and visualization. (Recall that, in a relaxed state, Natalie visualizes filling balloons with negative thoughts, dispersing the filled spheres into the universe, where they are neutralized so they won't return. [If you are a sci-fi enthusiast, perhaps identify the balloons as "alien transport vehicles!"] Alan visualizes bubbles like those formed by Alka-Seltzer Gold™.) Some patients visualize using a punching bag filled with anger or piercing the anger with darts, arrows, daggers, etc. Please note it is the anger you are destroying, not yourself or anyone else.

Immediate confrontation is an honest way to deal with anger directed at a friend or loved one, as long as he is grounded. As many body therapists suggest, let both sides deal with the anger, then kiss and make up, especially with your sleep partner. In an adverse situation with an employer or other authority figure, when confrontation is contraindicated, try an exercise that has benefited some of us. Stamp your feet, shake your legs and visualize dispersing your anger (or stamping it out) as you laugh and say aloud: "Excuse me, my foot has fallen asleep." Your laughter further reduces your internal tension and breaks down the anger barrier between you and your adversary.

---

[i] Ephesians (IV-14), King James Version.

Timing is Everything In whatever way you vent your anger (or other emotion), by subterfuge, confrontation or exercise, the least appropriate time is just before bedtime. Just before you go to sleep, appropriate breathing, grounding and relaxation improve the quality of sleep. Better sleep will eventually have a positive effect on your meditation technique.

PRACTICAL APPLICATIONS

♪♪♪♪♪

I use bedtime Meditation/Relaxation techniques to allow me to embrace positive suggestions. Alan discusses sleep in the context of energy. From our discussions about sleep, I have started using my aura in new ways. After a brief meditation, I play with my aura, sending energy from my fingertips to my CROWN Chakra, which encompasses the brain. I visualize the stream from my fingers acting as a tranquilizer. I feel the benefits without the need for over-the-counter or prescription drugs.

Example 1 When I have writer's block and struggle to find a way to express thoughts that I consider vital, I use methods described in Chapter 9 (Conditioning). Using the pattern of three, I repeat three times that my Mind/body/soul/spirit is clearing all frustrations, allowing me deep sleep. I impart the suggestion that in the morning I'll be wide awake and alert with a clear, fresh idea of ways to overcome my block. More often than not, I arise refreshed and ready to continue writing.

Example 2 When I have retired too late to get more than five of my required seven hours of sleep, I include in my meditation a suggestion of distorted time. I instill the suggestion that my Mind/body/soul/spirit will distort the five hours into a peaceful, restful energy usually acquired in seven hours. (The more often you practice, the sooner your body responds.)

Note that I said "my required seven hours of sleep." As with everything else, optimum sleep time is individual and variable. Once you have developed a positive sleep habit, your body will tell you what you need. Until I learned grounding and relaxation techniques, I used to be tired no matter how long I slept. Now after six and a half or seven hours – depending upon my Accordion Reserve©, I awaken refreshed and ready to tackle any and every problem.

Caution Use time distortion only occasionally when you don't have enough time to replenish your body with completely relaxed sleep. The procedure worked too well for one person; during a crisis, he punished his body by overuse of time distortion, resulting in lower resistance to infection.

Example 3 Just before I fall asleep, I check my clock for the time and suggest to myself that I wake fifteen minutes before the alarm will ring. Please note: Setting the alarm is particularly important to avoid negative thoughts intruding in dreams – like those that used to disturb my sleep: "I'll oversleep and miss my plane, be late for an appointment, be late for work."
♪♪♪♪

SUMMARY

To understand the effects of the ANS on sleep, refer to Chapter 6. In a nutshell, however, the parasympathetic nervous system (PSNS) promotes conservation and restoration of healing energy, while the SNS expends energy. Thus the ANS explains the need for relaxation techniques at bedtime (especially the need to practice developing proper breathing habits – see Chapter 7). By enhancing the PSNS, deep breathing creates a healing inner peace, while an agitated SNS disrupts sleep and healing.

The vagus nerve, the dominant parasympathetic nerve, controls most major organ functions. It stimulates the diaphragm to function more effectively, which, in turn, improves deep breathing.

Thus, utilizing visualization enhances vagal function, promotes PSNS performance, and heals Mind/body/soul/spirit.

FINAL VERSES

Positive Thinking In keeping with lessons of preceding chapters, restore positive thinking to your sleep even if you are already a good sleeper. There may be times when the following techniques will be helpful.

Prior to sliding under the covers, follow a simple sequence of behaviors that you associate with successful sleep. Terminate all chores, complete appropriate hygiene and settle into a passive, gentle wind-down activity such as reading poetry, reassuring religious texts or other non-provocative content.

You can also listen to peaceful music. Reinforcing our musical Accordion theme, we suggest several accordion recordings[i,ii] that enhance calming energy. As Pauline Oliveros[iii] writes: "The accordion has a wealth of overtones, dynamics, and it **breathes**." (Our emphasis. Note the connection with the PSNS and breathing.) Whenever we play "The Beauty of Sorrow"[2], listeners invariably experience a PSNS response. Positive conditioning promotes an uncluttered mind. Summon soothing experiences and sensations that you associate with a good night's sleep. Focus on one of these images as you use your relaxation techniques.

---

[i] Goldstein Gil. 1995. "Detour Ahead" (Frigo/Carter/Ellis). Big World Records from *The World According to Gil.* Reproduced on Disc 2, Track 4 in *Planet Squeezebox.* Ellipsis Arts… . Roslyn, NY.
[ii] Oliveros, Pauline. 1987. "The Beauty of Sorrow (excerpt)". Deep Listening Publications. Reproduced on Disc 2, Track 5 Ibid.
[iii] Oliveros, Pauline. 1995. *Planet Squeezebox.* p. 27.

14
NUTRITION –
Building Cell Energy

Prologue

"MANN IST WAS ER ISST" "One is what one eats" is philosopher Ludwig Feuerbach's[1] play on words, often quoted or paraphrased.

Diets are the staple of life. You can't live without eating. Today, with the emphasis on maintaining normal body weight, people are besieged with different approaches for losing weight. Everyone thinks he has the answer. There are those who advocate that all calories are the same. In other words, "Just eat less" is the typical "non-prescription" for overweight patients.

There are those who emphasize certain types of foods, certain patterns of eating and so on, with the expectation that following a particular approach (use your conditioning!) will help you reduce your body fat. In turn, that should help you prevent diabetes and heart disease. Obesity and weight loss are a public obsession. We obviously can't do justice to any one diet plan in this book, so we will provide reference resources to point you in the right direction to integrate diet, exercise, sleep and relationships into an Accordion-expanding, Environmental Health-building lifestyle.

Toxins and Overweight We have alluded to observations that many toxic exposures we encounter in daily living are fat-soluble. In other words, when your liver can't convert toxins to water-soluble forms for excretion in stool, urine, sweat and breath, toxins will tend to accumulate wherever there is fat. Depending on that site of deposition, symptoms may develop over time. If you are genetically predisposed to gain weight, your protection is to eat, thus making fat a "safe" reservoir to store toxins. That will protect you until your

151

pancreas can't keep up with the extra blood sugar that results from these eating patterns. That's when elevated blood pressure, diabetes and heart disease set in.

When you try to lose weight, the process works in reverse. Most diet plans do not include the provision to compensate for stored toxins in body fat. When you burn fat, stored toxins are released, placing an extra burden on your liver. If chemical pathways (enzymes) are ineffective because you are vitamin or mineral deficient, or inappropriate chemical signals are interfering, you may temporarily lose weight. When the factory (liver machinery) gives out, the residual release of toxins stimulates another round of eating to make more body fat. We hypothesize that toxin recycling undermines the success rate of most diet plans.

Toxins and Underweight While clearly in the minority, underweight people are just trying to build and maintain body weight. As a rule, as we all age, we tend to lose 10% of our muscle mass for each decade that we live beyond about age 40. If you can't digest, absorb, eat or tolerate nutrient-rich foods, then you too, are at serious risk of dumping toxins into your bloodstream and forcing your liver to work overtime. When you can't absorb nutrients, the liver sooner or later gives out (although it hangs on for an incredibly long time), and toxins distribute as they would when you diet or when you fast. Poor eating habits only exacerbate the problem. Fasting increases nausea, which leads to poor appetite, leading to muscle (internal protein source) breakdown, further burdening the liver.

Suboptimal Health In Chapter 5, we commented that you can live for a long time in "relatively good health" – which means that you may have a relatively expanded Accordion, slowly collapsing, but without any untoward symptoms. If this is you, then you belong to the "Silent Minority" of the apparently healthy. Then, all of a sudden, illness after illness sets in. The hypothesis for your condition is that in the absence of adequate supplementation to your diet, your liver eventually loses its ability to keep up with its daily activity to keep your Accordion expanded, and you become symptomatic.

VITAMINS AND MINERALS SERVE MULTIPLE FUNCTIONS

Science is slowly catching up with clinical observations of Environmental Medicine practitioners who for many years have espoused the importance of vitamin supplements.

The following topics are the basis for many textbooks, and we do not have the space or the expertise to delve into these topics in detail. We cover them briefly to illustrate how ample nutrients aid in expanding the Accordion Reserve© and improve the autonomic nervous system (ANS). In other words, they restore and redirect *Energy – the Essence of Environmental Health*.

Coenzymes - Enzyme Enhancers Biochemists long ago documented that enzymes cause chemical changes to occur at body temperature. Serving as coenzymes, vitamins and minerals improve enzyme function. Biochemists determine vitamins/mineral deficiencies by monitoring levels of enzyme-mediated chemical reactions.

Example 1 Vitamin B6 aids enzymes in more than 40 different chemical reactions ranging from sugar to essential fat to detoxication metabolism. In many of these same reactions, magnesium functions as a supplemental factor called a coenzyme.

Example 2 Vitamin C aids enzymes that process hormones, neurotransmitters, cholesterol and bile acids.

Nature's Scavengers Through natural, non-enzymatic pharmacologic mechanisms, larger quantities of vitamins and other nutrients (phytochemicals) act as antioxidants or scavengers to mop up debris from oxidation or acid buildup processes that occur in your body. This function of supplements is frequently overlooked when critics disparage large-dose vitamin supplementation.

SCAVENGERS, CHEMICAL PATHWAYS AND
THE AUTONOMIC NERVOUS SYSTEM

An important chemical pathway that processes toxins is called "methylation" (**ME**) (**Figure 14-1**). This pathway makes adrenalin, inactivates histamine, regulates neurotransmitters, repairs DNA, makes RNA and generates creatine.[2][3][4][5][6][7] In order for this reaction to proceed, your body needs a steady supply of methionine (**M**), an essential amino acid. After ME occurs, homocysteine (**HC**) is created. M can be reclaimed from HC, using folic acid (**FA**) and vitamin B12. Dr. Pall[8] postulated that B12 also functions as a scavenger for nitric oxide (**NO**), a neurotransmitter, made from arginine, which regulates pain and inflammation, blood vessel dilation and transport of sugar into muscle. FA scavenges for external sources of formaldehyde (**FO**), which is found in new wrinkle-free clothing, plywood and particle board, to name a few.[i] Linked to heart disease and stroke, elevated HC can also be lowered with vitamin B6 to make taurine (**T**) and glutathione (**G**).

Thus, HC is dangerous, until its level is lowered, by priming the ME pathway or making T and G. T acts as a scavenger to clean up chlorine products (like some pesticides and chlorinated organic matter found in tap water), provide energy to heart muscle and combine with cholesterol to make bile more liquid. G has many antioxidant scavenger functions, including processing solvents and

---

[i] Vinitsky A. 2004. *21st Century Miracle Treatment?*© (in press). Based on the scavenger principle, Dr. Vinitsky proposes that FA partners with B12 to recycle excess FO via ME. FO may be excessively produced inside your body when a neurotransmitter acetylcholine is metabolized instead of being taken up as it should be, by parasympathetic (PSNS) nerve endings. This scenario could occur when an over-functioning PSNS is attempting to turn off excess sympathetic nervous system (SNS) activity. Since FO has increased sympathetic activity, failure to reduce its level could cause prolonged SNS symptoms (see Chapters 6 and Professional Challenges). Additionally, he proposes that FA scavenges for glutamate (**GL**), an amino acid that is a component of FA itself. Thus, FA would function as a reservoir for GL. GL stimulates a receptor (N-methyl D-aspartate) that increases NO. Then very high levels of FA could lower pain and inflammation, allow for improved sugar transport to muscles (for more energy and lower risk of diabetes) and for arginine to be redirected to make creatine (energy source for brain cells, skeletal muscle and heart muscle). Finally, Dr. Vinitsky suggests that our bodies have a priority system for ME. Higher-ranked ME functions would be more active than lower ranking ones, which could be temporarily or permanently sacrificed. The ranking is: 1) adrenalin activation, 2) adrenalin inactivation, 3) histamine inactivation, 4) integration of norepinephrine, dopamine, serotonin and melatonin, 5) metabolism of hormones that look like adrenalin, 6) inactivating toxins, chemicals, niacin and medications, 7) repair of DNA and synthesis of RNA and 8) synthesis of creatine. He speculates that optimal health will occur only when there is sufficient FA and B12 available to cover all ME functions whenever needed.

acetaminophen, regulating B12 utilization in cells and reactivating vitamin C.

Therefore, it appears that if FA, B12, T and G are diverted for scavenger functions, there will be insufficient amounts of these to maintain proper energy for healing and repair. Lower priority ME reactions will be sacrificed.

Deficiencies can result in insomnia, injuries, high blood pressure, anxiety, depression, diabetes, high cholesterol, gallstones, hyperactivity, loss of memory and the "natural decline" in muscle mass during aging. In short, these "malfunctions" are a direct result of an overstressed, inflexible ANS.

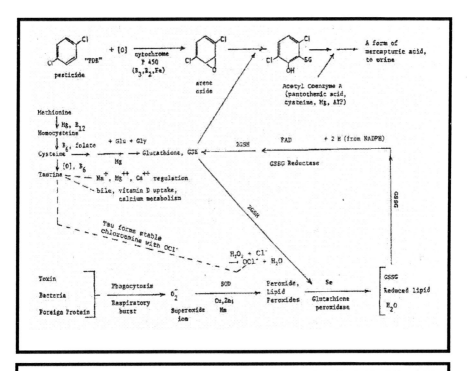

Figure 14-1. Methylation pathway. Diversion of vitamin B12, folic acid, taurine and glutathione to other chemical pathways may result in excess sympathetic stress. By permission from Bob Smith, Ph.D.)

If formaldehyde is involved in excess SNS activity (see previous footnote), then its presence may contribute to a weakened PSNS. And that in turn, is stress – a shrinking **Accordion Reserve©**.

SHRINKING ACCORDION RESERVE© –
OXIDATION AND ACID ACCUMULATION

There is potentially destructive energy flowing through your body as free radicals. These noxious particles are created when toxins interact with body tissue or when enzymes activate them in your cells.

Through a step-wise progression of energy transfer, oxidation-reduction reactions lower destructive energy so that it can be safely eliminated from your body or redirected for healing.

Oxidation and acidosis are both analogous to an over-stressed SNS. Oxidation/acidosis generates destructive and wasted energy in your body. Excess SNS activity also leads to energy expenditure. These destructive forces shrink the **Accordion Reserve©**.

Acid buildup (acidosis) is analogous to free radicals in its destructive energy force. Deep/rapid breathing serves as a rapid buffer system, resulting in a speedy elimination of carbon dioxide. A slower bicarbonate buffer system reverses the acid buildup for as long as possible. A gentle exercise program augments these processes by improving elimination of toxins through breathing, urination and stool/gas elimination.

Supplements and antioxidants ground your <u>destructive physical energy</u> in concert with your breathing. Acting like a lightning rod, conditioning, relaxation and meditation ground your <u>destructive emotional energy</u>. These countermeasures or treatments expand your **Accordion Reserve©**.

<u>*Safe Energy Management*</u> A visual analogy (imagery) can help you understand the progression of how antioxidants and buffers help protect you. Visualize boating over a falls. You'd capsize because of sudden energy transfer (from gravity and the force of the

water flowing). But travel down in a lock system, and you are transferred step-wise – safely and securely.

Nutrients and Commercial Food Sources In today's commercialized food delivery system, most food sources are processed, raised or grazed hastily and reaped prematurely. "Mass-produced" results in "mass delivery," causing nutrient-depleted food. Another consequence of mass food marketing is the need to preserve foodstuffs so that they have a longer shelf life. Additives and preservatives "enhance" and imitate flavors, add color and prevent wastage, but at a severe liability. These additives are residues which cause many individual sensitivities. **Bugs won't eat these treated foods. Why should we?**

When Is an Apple Really an Apple? Nutritional contents vary in the foods you eat – water, calories, vitamins and minerals. The contents depend on soil nutrients and available water supply. Unless food has been organically cultivated, the food you eat frequently acts as a transporter for hidden items such as man-made additives, preservatives or pesticides.

The histogram (**Figure 14-2**)[9] below illustrates the difference between organically grown vs. commercially grown foods. In general, there is a higher quantity of desirable nutrients (in this case minerals) and a lesser amount of contaminants (toxic metals) in organically grown food.

When you are planning your diet, include as much organic food as possible and check the necessary nutrients in order to build your cell energy.

A standard diet exposes you to more additives, preservatives and toxins, generating more free radicals. Your body is more willing to accept exposure to natural substances than to synthetics. Those which are recognized as synthetic must be processed for excretion. These materials become free radicals on their way to being excreted.

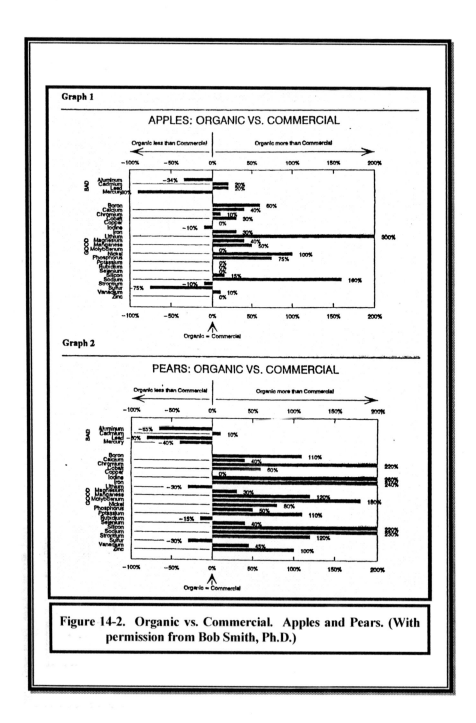

Figure 14-2. Organic vs. Commercial. Apples and Pears. (With permission from Bob Smith, Ph.D.)

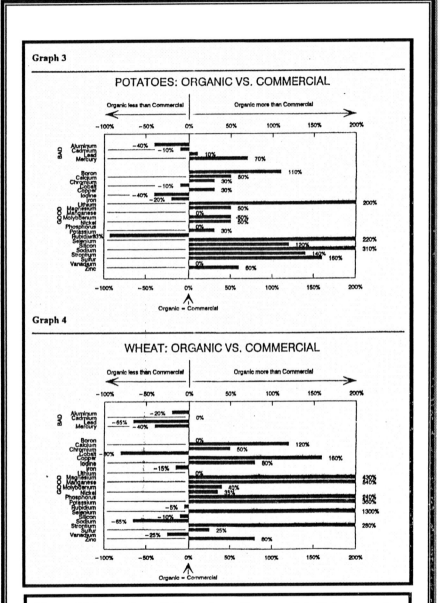

Graph 3

POTATOES: ORGANIC VS. COMMERCIAL

Graph 4

WHEAT: ORGANIC VS. COMMERCIAL

Figure 14-2. (continued) Organic vs. Commercial. Potatoes and
Wheat. (With permission from Bob Smith, Ph.D.)

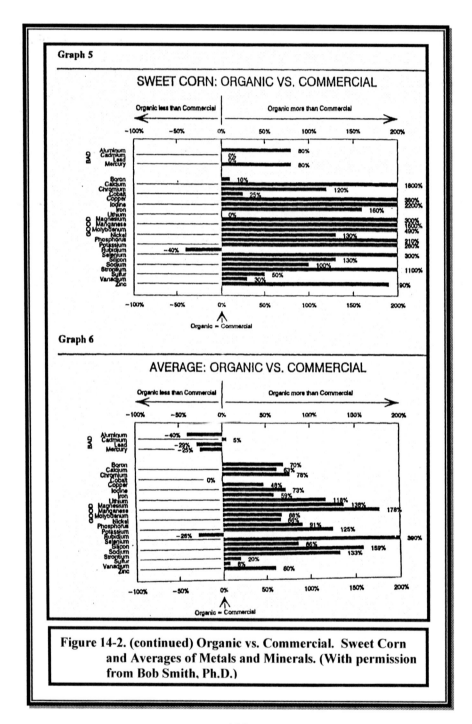

Figure 14-2. (continued) Organic vs. Commercial. Sweet Corn and Averages of Metals and Minerals. (With permission from Bob Smith, Ph.D.)

Thus, the standard diet potentially subjects you to a shrinking Accordion, impaired **Body Tolerance** and a stressed ANS.

Foods - Acid or Alkaline Refer to Appendix C, the table[10] which identifies foods by their tendency to make you alkaline or acid. Neutral pH is 7.0. Less than 7 is acid; more than 7, alkaline. Your body and tissue pH (acid level) is about 7.4. Therefore, you should be slightly alkaline.

Use Appendix C to help you determine if your diet is acid- or alkaline-forming. A preferred diet should be about 60% alkaline and 40% acid. If you are like most Americans, you probably eat many more acid-forming foods.

Adjusting your diet to a more favorable alkaline balance can help you expand your **Accordion Reserve©**, build your **Body Tolerance** of the environment and balance your ANS.

VARIETY - THE "SPICE OF LIFE"

Food Choices Limited food choices can result in:
*   Toxin accumulation – If conventional foods are repeat-edly chosen, pesticides and/or additives are present in larger quantities.
*   Nutritional deficiencies
    *   From a lack of intake.
    *   From wearing down enzyme pathways that de-pend on vitamins and minerals to maintain opti-mal performance. The vitamins are depleted from this excessive wear.

Therefore, **a goal of optimal nutritional and Environmental Health is to seek a varied sampling of foods in your diet.**

Rotation Diet If you are chemically sensitive, you no doubt have heard of a rotation diet. Natalie's *If This Is Tuesday, It*

Must Be Chicken taught many people how to prevent worsening sensitivities while maintaining an expanded variety of foods in their diets. Since *Chicken* is out of print and in the oven, her book with Dr. Rea, *Success in the Clean Bedroom,*[i] dispenses the same lesson.

EXERCISE AND NUTRITION

Exercise Sandwich If you think the Exercise Sandwich© is something to eat, you're in for a letdown. But read in Chapter 15 how you can plan a program to assist you in correcting your metabolism.

SUMMARY

Dr. Herb L. Tea[ii] offers the following "nutrition prescription":

* Eat lots of different foods.
* Savor foods for their flavor, color, texture, sound and aroma.
* Select organic foods whenever possible to reduce your daily intake of pesticides, additives, preservatives and manufactured hormones.
* Plan your diet with foods that promote better acid/alkaline balance.

---

[i] Available in limited supply. See our website www.alanrvinitskymd.com for details.

[ii] Whenever Alan decides to be "punny [sic]" Natalie laughs but wants you to know that she always quotes Samuel Johnson, who repeatedly said: "The pun is the lowest form of humor."

[1] Feuerbach L. *Das Geheimnis des Opfers,* 1864 (translated *The Secret of the Victim*).

[2] Walsh W. 1997. Biochemical treatment of mental illness and behavior disorders. Presented at the Minnesota Brain Bio Association. Available on the Health Research Institute website http://www.hriptc.org.

[3] Rosenblatt DS, Fenton WA. 2001. Inherited Disorders of Folate and Cobalamin Transport and Metabolism. In *The Metabolic & Molecular Bases of Inherited Disease*, 8th Ed., Scriver CR et al., eds. McGraw-Hill, New York, pp. 3897-3933.

[4] Bredt DS. Nitric Oxide Synthases. In *The Metabolic & Molecular Bases of Inherited Disease*, 8th Ed., Scriver CR et al., eds. McGraw-Hill, New York, pp. 4275-90.

[5] Waly M. Olteanu H, Banerjee R, Choi S-W, Mason JB, Parker BS, Sukumar S, Shim S, Sharma A, Benzecry JM, Power-Charnitsky V-A, Deth RC. 2004. Activation of methionine synthase by insulin-like growth factor-1 and dopamine: a target for neurodevelopmental toxins and thimerosal. *Molecular Psych* 9:358-70.

[6] Timonen M, Jokelainen J, Hakko H, Silvennoinen-Kassinen S, Meyer-Rochow VB, Herva A, Räsänen P. 2003. Atopy and depression: results from the Northern Finland 1966 Birth Cohort Study. *Molecular Psych* 8:738-44.

[7] Moretti A, Gorini A, Villa RF. 2003. Affective disorders, antidepressant drugs and brain metabolism. *Molecular Psych* 8:773-85.

[8] Pall ML. 2002. NMDA sensitization and stimulation by peroxynitrite, nitric oxide, and organic solvents as the mechanism of chemical sensitivity in multiple chemical sensitivity. *FASEB Jl* 16:1407-17.

[9] Smith R. Bionostics, Inc. (Reproduced with permission.)

[10] Jaffe R. "Food & Chemical Effects on Acid/Alkaline Body Chemical Balance." October 2002. (Reproduced with permission.)

15
MOVEMENT AND RHYTHM -
"No Sweat" Is a Problem

Prologue

The Hated "E" Word - EXERCISE Many people just hate to exercise! And you may be one of them, even if you are active in sports. In keeping with one of the themes of this book, it's time to turn those negative thoughts into positives. Overweight, out-of-shape physicians who don't exercise cannot teach you by example. However, unless a qualified person is willing to talk to you about exercise, you are probably not going to get really involved. Exercise is usually vaguely defined, if at all. An exercise "prescription" is non-existent, just like the nutrition "non-prescription" in the preceding chapter.

Unless you are decidedly motivated to be active, probably your last organized exercise participation was in high school. Some of you may be "weekend warriors," while others engage in team sports that may be recreational or cardiac and life enhancing. Since readers will likely be at different levels of fitness, the importance of this chapter is to emphasize some common features of exercise and advance what you've already accomplished.

LEARN FROM INFANTS

By watching a baby move you can perceive the meaning of exercise. Notice how an infant rhythmically moves arms and legs to sound and voice, eventually does partial push-ups, rolls over, pulls legs to chest, sits up, crawls, pulls up, walks, climbs, runs and jumps. These are all large muscle movements, which come naturally in development. This sequence emphasizes flexibility of the trunk and its limb attachments at the shoulders and hips. At any level of fitness, we should all strive to accomplish similar goals.

Turn on some pleasant, relaxing music or sing your own. Remember to breathe deeply or practice **Relaxation Breathing** during each exercise.

* Move your arms and legs.
* Step in place.
* March to the rhythm.
* Move your legs side to side.
* Circle your arms forward and backward.

♫♫♫♫♫

If you are wheelchair bound, you can still do the same! (Some of my diabetic patients have been observed to get up and walk again after initiating this program!)
♫♫♫♫♫

* Now advance to your torso.
* Bend to your sides.
* Twist at your hips by turning your shoulders.
* Rotate your body in circles to the left and to the right.

<u>Comment</u> Just as your arm or leg is attached at a rotating joint, your torso is attached at the pelvis by a flexible pole – your spine. This program is a good warm-up for more advanced athletes and essential for chronically ill patients.

TO GET YOURSELF GOING, IMAGINE YOURSELF AS AN INFANT

* Lying on your back, using one leg or both, rhythmically pull your knees to your chest.
* Lift your shoulders off the floor.
* Twist your shoulders side to side.
* Twist your hips side to side.
* Roll over to each side.
* Get on your belly and do partial pushups with knees on floor.

* Get on your hands and knees and rock forward and back.
* Arch your back up and pull it down.

RHYTHMIC MOVEMENT

♫♫♫♫♫

Think what you've just accomplished. It's rhythmic movement! It's simple and easy, nothing more than my baby patient needs to do to prepare himself for the more rigorous movements of crawling, pulling up, walking, climbing and running that follow.
♫♫♫♫♫

A Good Beginning You just did it with little motivation! If a baby can do it, so can you! In exercise terms, you just accomplished a lot — warming your muscles and promoting flexibility through repetition of muscle groups. You are preparing for more "work" ahead. And you did it with minimal effort. Build on this positive experience. Grow into the feeling of movement.

Try to start this routine about 15 minutes after each meal. Linking movement with eating has many virtues, the most important of which is to reduce peak blood sugar after a meal. This is by far one of the best methods to prevent and/or treat diabetes.

♫♫♫♫♫

Exercise Sandwich Our mothers' childhood advice, "don't go swimming after you eat; you'll get a cramp," will encourage you to eat smaller portions if you plan to move soon after. (See how you just turned negative thinking into positive motivation.) Remember – you can always eat again when you finish moving. In fact, that's a good idea, giving your body a chance to recover more quickly from the movement. That's what I call the Exercise Sandwich©, when the duration and intensity of your activity increase. (See **Figure 15-1.**)

Once you are finally moving regularly and rhythmically, you can advance to the next level. Remember – it feels good to move, especially if you ease into it! At this stage, you'd like your movement to promote additional gains.

167

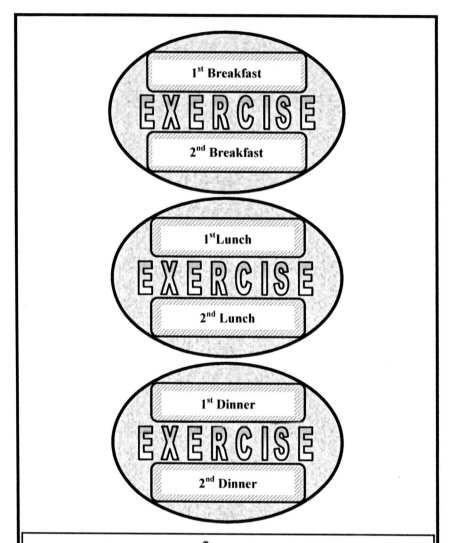

Figure 15-1. **The Exercise Sandwich**©. Ideally 3 pairs of meals with exercise simulate contemporary hunter-gatherer diet. Carbohydrate utilization during exercise minimizes insulin stimulation. Insulin resistance can be bypassed; weight loss is encouraged.

      Adapted from The Zone Diet,[H] adequate protein, fat and carbohydrates primarily from vegetable and fruit sources. A large variety of foods, such as the rotation diet, is discussed in Chapter 17.

[H]Sears, B. *The Zone, A Dietary Road Map*, Harper Collins Publishers, Inc., New York, 1995, and its updates.

THE CAT

I discovered a comfortable position to begin stretching exercises. I previously learned this position in teaching patients how to care for their backs.

"The cat" seemed like an appropriate introduction to exercise because the position reminded me of infants during their physical development. I explored the sensations that resulted from moving my back in a rhythmic pattern.

Then Natalie taught me effective breathing techniques. Gradually we improved upon the breathing technique and eventually related the combined movement, breathing, and relaxation to our work with the autonomic nervous system (ANS). You can do the same - combine lessons from various chapters and mold them into your own techniques.

THE CAT AS I KNOW IT

As you begin this and subsequent exercises, if necessary, refresh your memory by referring to the section in Chapter 7 on Developing PSNS Breathing Pattern.

* Get on "all fours."
* Gently breathe in and out slowly for 3 seconds (normal uncontrolled breathing is PSNS Breathing).
* Make your lower back curve by pushing your abdomen towards the floor, while elevating your head (*Lower Back Stage*).
* Bear down and push. Hold breath for 3 seconds.
* Slowly exhale, lowering your head (PSNS Breathing).
* Reposition back to neutral position for 3 seconds, breathing gently in and out (uncontrolled PSNS Breathing).
* While raising upper back toward the sky, take a full breath in through your mouth like a yawn, filling lungs completely as if they were balloons, and hold for 3 seconds. Also elevate your head (Deep Breathing Stage).
* Slowly exhale, lowering your head (PSNS Breathing).

169

* Return to neutral position for 3 seconds, breathing gently (PSNS Breathing).
* Alternately repeat *Lower Back/Deep Breathing Stages* 3 times.

EXERCISE CONDITIONING

Five "P's" Condition yourself for Planning, Preparation, Perseverance, Perception and Patience. Above I mentioned planning movement and linking it to eating. This is conditioning at its best.

A successful program has an outline, format, objective and outcome. To accomplish these, you <u>plan</u> and <u>prepare</u>. Fortunately, once you are conditioned to do these as part of your improved lifestyle, the time for planning and preparation will be markedly reduced.

Stick with your plan; the positive conditioning and good feeling when you move will help you <u>persevere</u>. In time, you will apply <u>perception</u> – your Body Awareness – to your program. <u>Patience</u> will be needed because observable improvements come slowly over time. Therefore, tailor your long-term expectations into short-term objectives and goals that are easily achievable. For example: "Today I will do additional movements linked to eating twice. Tomorrow I will do them three times."
♫♫♫♫♫

GOAL-ORIENTED 5 P'S

The following illustrates how you can gradually improve your exercise conditioning:

* "I can do movement 5 minutes, and I get tired.
* I would like to do 6 minutes.
* I will try 3 minutes, take a break for 3 minutes, then try 3 minutes again.
* (Accomplish this and you have now completed 6 minutes!)
* Next time, I will try it with only a 2-minute break, and the time after that, only a 1-minute break. Finally I will do 6 minutes without a break."

Repetition for Emphasis The above simple sequence of thinking involves planning, preparing, persevering, perceiving and patience. There is a <u>short-term goal</u> of a shorter rest period between movements that are not as lengthy and a <u>longer-term goal</u> of increasing movement for only 1 minute more without tiring.

Making your goals achievable is crucial to feeling successful and reinforcing your daily movement. These concepts, incidentally, are adaptable to all lifestyle changes.

Exception The short-term goal in the example above suggested making your goal a tiny bit harder (in this case, a shorter rest period between the 3-minute movement). However, sometimes you need an easy day or a different activity as an additional recovery time. People who are used to exercising may get compulsive or too intense about it, and they eventually injure themselves. If you find yourself in this situation, a suitable goal might be:

*   "I'm going to go as slowly as I can today," or
*   "I'm only going to stretch today" or
*   "I'm going to rest today."

Caution This concept of a "rest goal" applies to individuals who have already gone to the other extreme, i.e., those who are already "conditioned" to excess and those who frequently suffer injuries. Excess is as potentially dangerous as is the extreme of not being active.

LARGER, LONG-TERM GOALS

Why Exercise at All? What are you hoping to accomplish? One or more of the following objectives will influence your short-term goals:

*   Maintain health.
*   Rehabilitate one or more injured body parts.

* Lose weight.
* Improve flexibility.
* Gain strength.
* Increase metabolism.
* Participate or become competitive in a particular sport.
* Detoxify (getting rid of stored chemicals, usually in body fat, membranes or organs).

<u>*Detox*</u> Detoxifying is a singularly important goal because it expands your **Accordion Reserve**©.[i] Commonly we think of "detoxing" in terms of alcohol or drugs. However, to maintain health your body is in a constant protective posture by "detoxing" all types of pollution. Your exercise program enhances your body's ability to achieve that goal.

ADVANTAGES - TO YOUR HEALTH

Exercise:
* Increases heat production, and sweating promotes body cooling.
* Increases blood flow to lungs, muscles, body fat, kidneys and liver.
* Increases fat burning and release of toxins dissolved in fat.
* Hastens elimination of toxins by increasing breathing rates and exchange of toxins from blood to expired air.
* Increases metabolism to convert toxins to water-soluble form for excretion in bile and urine.
* Improves energy utilization and organ system efficiency over time, i.e. increases the **Accordion Reserve**©.
* Increases sympathetic nervous system (SNS) activity during more vigorous exercise.

---

[i] Refer to the Glossary to understand the distinction between a program to "detox" and what your body does to "detox."

* Promotes healing by stimulating the PSNS as a response to the increase of SNS activity (see Chapter 3, "Alan's Story").
* Promotes PSNS activity during steady gentle exercise.

Caution Extremes of exercise or non-exercise pose undesirable consequences to health. Exercise is a graduated program for healing. Intense exercise when your body is not prepared for it may result in serous injury.

SWEATING

Exercise promotes your body's ability to clear toxins by sweating. Sweating is one of several ways to eliminate toxins from your body.[i] If your sweat has an unpleasant odor, don't reach for the deodorant, start exercising. You are eliminating toxins from your body! Even if you are not obviously sweating and have BO, bacteria in the skin and sweat glands of your armpits have created the bad odor from the chemicals you are excreting.

Society learned the art of covering up bad odors with more "pleasant" but toxic scents (perfumes) and suppressing our sweat production. Neither of these is desirable when you are considering "detoxing."

DISORDERS OF SWEATING

You can sweat excessively, at inappropriate times or from localized parts of your body or not at all. Excessive sweating can cause dehydration, while inappropriate sweating may be an inconvenience or an embarrassment (e.g. BO, cold hands) or a topic of conversation (Alan has been observed to sweat profusely from the neck up when he eats ethnic foods flavored with chili peppers!) Lack of sweating can result in body tissues overheating or contribute to build-up of toxins.

---

[i] Generalized sweating is a PSNS response. Localized sweating of the hands, for example, is an SNS response.

173

The inappropriate extremes of sweating represent a malfunction of the ANS and require medical attention. Correcting inappropriate sweating coincides with healing the ANS.

HEAT EXHAUSTION and HEAT STROKE are serious complications of exposure to high ambient temperatures and humidity. Because extreme dehydration has developed, the body cannot tolerate further fluid depletion. The sweat mechanism turns off, and normal sweating stops. "Gooseflesh" is the first sign of these emergency, life-threatening conditions. Immediate cooling is required.

WHY SWEAT?

Since you can never totally avoid all toxins, it makes sense to utilize all of your available mechanisms to eliminate them from your body. Usually it is only the sweat mechanism that requires your active encouragement.

Making Sweat, Drinking Water If you're "healthy," then you're probably sleeping, eating, coping and exercising effectively. (Healthy and symptom-free do not mean the same thing, however!) Vigorous activity can help you sweat and eliminate some of the pollutants of daily exposure. Even if you don't normally sweat from casual exercise or if you are not yet physically fit to engage in intense exercise, you can add layers of clothing to increase your body temperature and induce sweating. Drinking plenty of pure water before, during and after exercise enhances sweating. Larger volumes of water also protect against dehydration and muscle cramping. Starting to exercise with a water surplus is desirable. However, like anything done to an extreme, massive increases in water consumption are potentially toxic.

Sweating as Therapy If you are ill from any of a variety of conditions that result from toxic overload, then you can actually engage in a program that helps you eliminate toxins from your body.

Increased sweating is part of the plan. You can induce sweating as described above.

Additional treatments to promote sweating include niacin and a mineral bath or sauna to follow the exercise activity. Since this technique requires careful medical supervision, the details have been omitted. In addition, if you have ANS dysfunction with low blood pressure symptoms, such therapy is usually contra-indicated. (Warning signs you see on steam baths and saunas at health spas and fitness centers are actually highlighting conditions that are associated with changes of the ANS!)

SWEATING CONCLUSIONS

Sweating:
* Is an important body mechanism to lower excess body temperature and to eliminate toxins.
* Eliminates excess fluid secondarily.
* Excesses cause dehydration and a sense of feeling chilled.
* Excesses may result from a very large muscle mass, elevated body temperature, elevated ambient temperature, toxicity from or sensitivity to chemicals, medications or other substances.
* Absence may be abnormal and is life threatening if it develops during prolonged heat exposure.
* Is an important clue in assessing your ANS.

RECOGNIZING TOXIC OVERLOAD

Sweating is a major clue for detecting toxic overload. In most other respects, you may feel symptom-free, but not necessarily healthy. You may also be confusing "just the way you are" with a lack of symptoms. (Remember: a child doesn't realize he has poor vision until he gets glasses.)

Symptoms of Toxic Overload:
* Compulsive need to exercise

* Deteriorating or absent sense of smell
* Odor sensitivity and highly sensitive olfactory sense (especially cigarette smoke and perfumes)
* Irritable senses for stressful situations, light, sound, taste, touch, balance and coordination
* Fluctuating mood, concentration or memory depending on your environment
* Irregular bowel habits accompanied by indigestion or excess gas
* Aching, swollen joints or muscles
* Unexplained fluctuating fatigue
* Unexplained and erratic skin rashes
* Asthma and/or multiple allergies

You may recognize that symptoms of toxic overload are equivalent to dysfunction of the ANS.

SUMMARY

Plan, prepare, perceive, persevere and patiently perform:

* Progressive movement – rhythmically and regularly, like a baby who prepares for more advanced activity.
* Movement linked to eating – providing conditioning and consistency.
* Goal-oriented activities that promote daily, weekly and long-term success.

Movement and sweating reciprocally expand your **Accordion** Reserve©. Movement functions on the Energy Handle of the Accordion. Sweating (detoxing) functions on the Environmental Handle. As you detox, you improve coordination, which improves exercise, which improves detox, and so on…

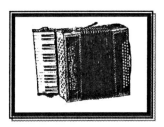

16

IMPROVING AIR QUALITY
- Breath of Life -
Little Things Mean a Lot!

Prologue

Unless you live in a "bubble," it is impossible to avoid all toxic exposures in today's living conditions. We advocate that you substitute less toxic products and increase your Accordion Reserve© with energy and safe environmental techniques.

♫♫♫♫

I participated in a task force mandated by Congress and executed by Federal Health Agencies.[1] When the group (leaders of medical and health organizations and health agencies) divided into four sections, we met in smaller poorly ventilated meeting rooms of a motel in suburban Washington. My section was asked to discuss "how to educate the public about the dangers of poor air quality."

The moderator (an M.D.) wrote each participant's suggestion on a large pad, tore off the sheets and posted them on the walls around the room. I began to recognize noticeable signs of participants' reactions. When it was my turn, I suggested that we prepare a list of common household toxic products like the moderator's magic marker that filled the room with toxic toluene fumes.

Many participants later admitted to me that they were uncomfortable (noticeably reacting) but never associated the discomfort with toxic fumes. One colleague commented to me, "How can we educate the public if we are so uninformed about the little things that are so troublesome?"

The next day, the moderator made a point of showing me that he had substituted water-based magic markers. The moderator turned a negative into a positive. He improved air quality by taking two steps:

* Substituting a less toxic product
* Opening the doors

Little things mean a lot!

(Please note that these participants were "healthy." They appeared to have a relatively good Accordion Reserve©. At best, some patients who suffer from Environmentally Triggered Illness [ETI] must use a mechanical metal pencil to write. Frequently they become ill from a wood pencil, a pen and most definitely a magic marker.)

♪♪♪♪

SENSITIVITY VS TOXICITY

Sensitivity to the environment must be distinguished from toxicity. "Safe levels" of chemicals are often quoted as standard guidelines. "Safe levels" apply to toxicity of substances only. (For example, there is no safe level for molds.) Exposure above safe levels should result in a statistical number of individuals developing the same reactions. However, sensitivity is a very individual response. For example, not everyone who smokes cigarettes gets lung cancer.

If you are constantly exposed to toxins in air, food or water, and these accumulate in your body, new sensitivities can develop.[2] Individual responses, genetic predisposition and variable symptoms make sensitivity hard to quantify and identify.

As described in Chapter 5, individual responses confound our best medical scientists because classical statistical analysis seldom reveals confirmation necessary to skeptics' satisfaction. Thus, sensitivity is reported as "anecdotes" – individual case reports which are relegated to less well-known medical publications. This information is no less important or less meaningful.

What is lacking is an improved method for analyzing data. However, the Accordion Reserve© model reminds scientists to include multiple variables in evaluating their hypotheses.

You yourself may be an anecdote and not know how you became one. No one is truly safe. Even if you are a well-conditioned athlete, your defenses may be susceptible to breakdown following prolonged training or intense competition. The results may initially present as recurrent infections, injuries or fatigue.

If You Have ETI - Don't Panic!

Educate, Strengthen and Protect:
* Learn which toxins cause or add to your health problems.
* Learn from success stories of Environmental Medicine (EM) practitioners and countless ETI sufferers who conquered their problems.
* Strengthen your immune and autonomic nervous systems.
* Protect yourself from toxic exposures that are a constant threat.
* Choose steps to preserve or improve your health.

The Allergic Masses

Sufferer You know or think you know you have allergies when you suffer from:
* Stuffy, drippy or runny nose
* Itchy, bloodshot eyes
* Rashes, including hives
* Asthma
* Sinus headaches
* Sudden swollen lips
* Red, hot ears

Relief You seek relief by:
* Trekking to your doctor for your perennial allergy shot
* Trying all the brands of over-the-counter and prescription "allergy and sinus" medications – hoping that one will help more than the last one (much to your surprise, the ingredients are usually the same)
* Shopping for cures – doctor after doctor
* Rushing to the emergency room or urgent care center

Awareness Do you recognize yourself from the symptom or relief lists above? If so, you are probably a member of one of these groups:
* Health-conscious readers – uncertain if you have allergies
* Confirmed allergy patients – no doubts about your allergy status
* Undiagnosed but chronically symptomatic patients – with probable ETI, but need a health care provider to make the diagnosis
* Severe environmental reactors – for whom there is no doubt

Become aware of your potential to prevent, control and manage your allergies and sensitivities! It's more than just treating the symptoms.

SYMPTOM RELIEF VS. CURE

Symptoms Are Warnings Heed your symptoms. Listen to your body. The message may be cryptic, but with the help of the **Accordion Reserve**©, you can assist your practitioner in discovering the cause.

Symptom-relieving Therapies Symptom relief restores temporary function, but relief is not necessarily a cure. If the cause of the symptoms has been identified and the appropriate treatment applied, then relief may be a cure.

Multiple Symptoms, Multiple Causes In some instances, symptoms may be attributable to multiple causes. The model of the Accordion Reserve© clearly illustrates this concept. Therefore, multiple treatments may be required.

Ineffectiveness of Symptom Relief For chronic symptoms, symptom relief therapies may become ineffective. More potent remedies are then substituted to treat an upward spiral of symptoms, followed by another round of therapies.

Adverse Effects Treatments of any type can result in adverse symptoms. Sometimes, potent therapies may result in more severe side effects. Most unfortunate is the presence of adverse effects, while the cause of the condition is left unanswered.

Medicines as Symptom Relievers Antihistamines and decongestants sometimes relieve nasal drip of allergy and rhinitis, just as aspirin "treats" the pain and inflammation of arthritis. Neither treatment is regarded as a cure.

Take Charge of Your Health

About Allergy Shots Allergy immunotherapy is just a "shot in the arm." Any health care practitioner will confirm that an allergy shot is not a substitute for cleaning up the dust and mold in your living space. You must take charge and help yourself get well. There is so much that you can do to alleviate your reactions and avoid future problems. That is the message of this book.

Environmental Stress The Environmental Handle of the Accordion Reserve© identifies biologic, chemical and physical triggers. EM practitioners teach that modern synthetic chemicals are perhaps the most stress-producing factors of our environment. Alan's motto is: "A substance of exposure is no different from a substance of abuse."

Manufacturer Propaganda Media advertising influences public demand for products. Wrinkle-free and other synthetic materials made from petroleum by-products offer convenience, attractiveness, sex appeal, etc. The list of products is virtually endless. Every day you'll hear an ad for medications.

Do a little test. Next time you watch TV, listen to the commercials. Record how many relate to cosmetics, air fresheners and cleaners. Then add to these products such as paints, glues, insecticides and many more. You will never hear that these same products offgas. Vapors such as formaldehyde and volatile organic chemicals contribute to the contamination of our air.

However, by Food and Drug Administration (FDA) law you are required to hear a litany of side effects from pharmaceuticals. Did you ever wonder why there are so many side effects, and why they can be contradictory? Look no further than the autonomic nervous system, and you will discover the answer.

Olfactory Challenge - Your Nose Knows Best "Follow your nose" down supermarket lane. Test your **Body Awareness** for your reactions to the odors. Do you notice any change in the way you feel as you stand near the soaps and dishwasher compounds? No matter how slight the sensation, "little things mean a lot." Your exposure can be a small negative challenge to your **Accordion Reserve**©.

Olfactory Fatigue Pause in the same aisle. See how long it takes for the slight change in your sensations to disappear. Your **Accordion Reserve**© is compensating. Hang around a little longer. Did you find that the odor is less noticeable and eventually disappears from your awareness? Your olfactory fatigue has set in. While you may not be aware of the smell, the effects on your body may accumulate, depending on your detox mechanisms.

Silent Illness In the Foreword to *Coping with Your Allergies*,[3] Dr. Randolph wrote of suffering patients wondering: "How did I suddenly get into this fix?"

Most people ignore the significance of their olfactory warning. The less offensive the odor becomes, the more they think, "Everything is O.K." Time and again, we hear the sorry tales of patients who just had to get the job done. And they did – the job was themselves.

Your Choice - Now or Later Noxious substances take their toll even when you cannot detect them. As for avoiding pollutants, the acutely ill have no choice. At great cost, they must avoid everything that makes them ill. All other people with mild allergy and/or sensitivity to toxic products have a clear choice: simple prevention now or possibly drastic measures later. In any case, the treatment should not be worse than the disease. The transition can be at your own pace, as long as you recognize that there is preventive value in acting sooner than later.

SUBSTITUTIONS - GRADUAL CHANGE

Anticipate If you have not already done so, this is a good time to start developing sound environmental habits. These little changes do not require major adjustments in your lifestyle. Take note of the continuous repetition of "little things mean a lot." No matter how minor, each avoidance or toxic exposure reduction results in an increase in your **Accordion Reserve**©. When avoidance is not possible, use your energy healing techniques (Chapters 7–12).

Personal Care Supplies Little things mean a lot. Choose to use:
* Unscented bath soaps, shampoos, cosmetics and deodorants
* Natural toothpaste
* No perfume, cologne or toilet water

Paper Products Little things mean a lot. Reduce exposure to formaldehyde, chlorine, dioxins and other toxins found in paper. Choose to use:
* Unscented, non-chlorinated white facial tissue and bathroom tissue paper

* Cotton towels instead of paper towels
* Cotton diapers instead of the disposable brands

Laundry and Cleaning Supplies Little things mean a lot. Scents, chlorine and ammonia add to the toxic burden. Choose to use:
* Unscented laundry soaps and fabric softeners, borax and baking soda
* Unscented and non-toxic cleaners, such as vinegar, and avoid ammonia, chlorine bleach and pine- and lemon-scented products

Fabrics When purchasing any fabric apparel, read both sides of the label. Frequently you will find 100% cotton on one side and a note on the other side indicating a percentage of polyester "on the facing." Little things mean a lot. Choose to use:
* Clothing made from natural fibers, such as cotton, wool, linen and silk
* A blend with at least 60% cotton
* Untreated fabrics (without mothproofing and wrinkle-free additives)
* Less toxic synthetic fibers; that is, choose nylon, Dacron and polyester in that order, but only as a last resort

Putting on a Party Substitute safely. Choose to:
* Use a hot tray to keep foods warm, and avoid using Sterno flames or candles
* Decorate with flowers, fruits or vegetables
* Use unscented candles made of beeswax instead of paraffin or preferably, none at all.

Purchases Check labels on all purchases. Little things mean a lot. Choose to use:
* "Less toxic products"
* Products with less odor
* Liquid sprays, rather than aerosols; "hypoallergenic" usually means synthetic and therefore, products so labeled usually are not acceptable

* A shower filter that reduces chlorinated organic matter from volatilizing

When Your Old Items Wear Out Select less toxic products. Choose to:
* Purchase cooking dishes made of Corning Ware, porcelain, stainless or enamel baked on cast iron, and when possible, avoid Bakelite handles, aluminum and Teflon coating
* Redecorate, renovate or build with nontoxic furnishings, upholstery, paints, construction materials, etc., many of which are less costly than similar products that are toxic

MOLD AND MILDEW

Mold and mildew present a serious cleaning problem for most everyone. Moisture and darkness invite mold growth. Damp, humid climates are fertile fields for mold. When indoor air dries and warms, some molds form spores. Condensation on windowpanes is a favorite site for mold growth. Molds also generate waste products that are toxic, including volatile organic chemicals and mycotoxins. If you are allergic/sensitive to mold, or affected by mold growth, the following are necessary for improving your indoor air quality.

PREVENTION

Main Concepts:
* Eliminate Danger zones:
    * Reduce moisture!!!
    * Caution:
        * Humidifiers and dehumidifiers are mold incubation systems.
        * Indoor plants and dried vegetation are indoor mold traps.
    * Keep area well ventilated and relatively warm, dry and well lit.
    * Leaks or floods: Use a portable electric heating unit to dry out and warm the area. Only if

absolutely necessary, use a dehumidifier to collect floodwater in the shortest time possible. Note caution above.

* Storage bins and hampers should be arranged to reduce moisture accumulation. Consider open net bags that can ventilate. Choose towel racks made from ceramic or chrome.
* Wooden portable clothes rack may be useful to condense drying areas.
* Fit shower stalls with glass doors.
* Use Barrier cloth[i] rather than vinyl for shower curtains (important provision for mold- and plastic-sensitive individuals).

* Destroy mold during air filtration – If you are not sensitive to electromagnetic radiation, you can add UV light attachments to air-handling systems or portable air filters.[ii]
    * Daily maintenance:
        * Wipe down shower, tub, basin and all floors in the bathroom after each use.
        * Hang towels, washcloths, bath mats and wipes to promote rapid drying. When possible wash them promptly, dry them quickly or both. Don't store in bins and hampers.
        * Store wet clothing in an open, well-ventilated space and process for washing/drying within 24 hours.
    * Weekly maintenance or more often:
        * Clean with vinegar, borax, diluted benzalkonium chloride, Rugged Red™ [iii]

---

[i] Barrier cloth is available from Janice's – proceed with caution – under new management. See Appendix D.
[ii] DUST-FREE 1-800-447-1100. Model AX-350 - with UV. See Appendix D.
[iii] Palmer Industries, Inc. See Appendix D.

or a chlorine-free, ammonia-free deter-
gent.
* Vinegar applied to a refrigerator door seal
can inhibit mold growth.
* Sprinkle dry borax or baking soda as a
deodorant and drying agent.
* Use a calcium chloride moisture trap.
Empty accumulated water.
* Drain sump pump of accumulated water.

* Indoor vigilance:
  * Identify and repair cracks in grout, tiles and
  walls, where moisture has a tendency to accumulate.
  * Consider sealing interior foundation walls
  with a relatively non-toxic product.[i]
  * Inspect pipe fittings, faucets and seals. Special attention should be directed at hidden areas such as under vanities and kitchen sinks.
  Repair leaks promptly.
  * Inspect for hard water mineral build-up in
  showers and tubs.
  * Turn off main water supply to the house when
  going on vacation. Leaks tend to occur during non-use because pressure builds up in the
  system.
  * Prevent pipe freezes during winter.

* Outdoor vigilance:
  * Identify and repair exterior cracks in and
  along rooflines, headers, fascia boards, cross-
  beams, crickets and skylights.
  * Free gutters of leaves and other vegetation to
  prevent water overflow.

---

[i] Palmer Industries, Inc. See Appendix D.

* Maintenance of yard should include cleaning and removing fallen leaves.

* Foundation should be inspected for water backflow. Soil should slope away from foundation.

BORAX - A SPECIAL FRIEND

Borax is a natural, sweet-scented mineral that is used in many cleaning products. A natural bleach and mold retardant, pure borax can be effective as an all-purpose cleaner. In a letter to Natalie, the late Dr. Lawrence D. Dickey, an EM pioneer, wrote this about borax:

"For almost ten years, between March 1966 and December 31, 1975, I carried out a hospital comprehensive environmental control program in evaluating patients with ecologic illness. This was accomplished in rooms made as chemically clean as possible. In addition to fixtures and furnishings that were free of plastics and other materials that were known to 'gas out,' the cleaning compounds were restricted to borax and filtered water. From February 15, 1972 on, the program was carried on in four especially constructed rooms with their own air-conditioning system separate from the rest of the hospital. This was the Poudre Valley Memorial Hospital Environmental Care unit. Control of chemical contaminates was much easier in this unit.

"Bacterial contamination in the past has been a problem in hospitals, and in ours, like others, the pathology department would periodically run culture checks in various areas of the hospital. The hospital pathologist found the rooms we used and the unit never failed any of their routine checks. We felt this very significant since none of the potent phenolic antiseptics were used in our area that were used in the rest of the hospital. It was a common observation that patients often had an adverse chemical reaction if they had occasion to leave the unit and enter the hospital proper.

"Borax is good deodorant, mold retardant and evidently a good bacteriostatic agent."

BENZALKONIUM CHLORIDE [i]

♪♪♪♪

I was given a freezer that became contaminated with mold. A friend cleaned that freezer using benzalkonium chloride, 17% strength, diluting one ounce in a gallon of water, making a final strength of 1/750. It took three washings with that strength and airing for a week after each washing, but after three weeks I gained the use of that freezer and had it for 15 years.

Caution ETI patients may require someone else to apply the benzalkonium chloride, then allow the space to offgas, to minimize reactions.

NATALIE'S NUGGETS

When we were stranded in the Metropolitan D.C. area without a doctor knowledgeable in ETI, our small support group survived by sharing homemade remedies to replace toxic products we could not tolerate.

We devised substitutes for toxic remedies for cleaning, for food recipes, for anything that made life easier. To demonstrate how you can do the same, I share with you cleaning hints that we used in a column called *Natalie's Nuggets.*

Vinegar Vinegar is an excellent mold retardant, especially when combined with borax. In my earlier books, I recommended vinegar to clean washing machines, dishwashers and for general housework.

When combined with borax, vinegar worked wonders in toilet and shower grooves and moldy corners in bathrooms and kitchens.

---

[i] Palmer Industries, Inc. See Appendix D.

For people sensitive to vinegar, we found substitutes:
* Granular vitamin C with borax for cleaning mold
* Baking soda on a warm surface of the stove or pots and pans (with a little vitamin C or lemon juice).
* Lemon juice instead of vinegar for recipes like mayonnaise as well as for cleaning

Experiment; use your own creativity.

By popular request from readers of my previous books, until further notice, <u>Natalie's Nuggets</u> will appear on our website.[4]

♪♪♪♪♪

OZONATOR - SAVIOR OR DESTROYER[i]

Depending on the severity of the pollution, an ozonator can sometimes be useful for removing mold and toxic chemicals.

Ozonator Specifications That Minimize Adverse Outcomes
* Timer – in working order
* Adjustable volume control – to set output to match volume of the treated space
* Concentration control

CAUTION Be certain that the machine is in excellent condition, use a distributor you trust, have the instructions in written form and follow the instructions exactly unless your health care provider offers other suggestions.

Safe Use to Prevent Disaster:
* Use a timed application of ozone. Better to apply two short treatments than to over-apply one.
* Seal the treated space from the remainder of the house.
* Crack open one window for ventilation.

---

[i] See Needs, Inc., Appendix D, for reliable information on purchasing ozonators.

* Vacate the house during timed application.
* Allow the unit to shut off for 1 hour or more before returning to the treated room.
* Ventilate treated space with fan and open windows after treatment is complete.

OZONE DISASTER ALERT – Over-treating with ozone can release embedded toxins from upholstery, carpets, walls, wallpaper and paint. The oxidation effects of ozone then convert these liberated chemicals to "free radicals." Inhaled, these free radicals are a disaster of the first degree.

SYNTHETIC CARPETS

The best advice we have for synthetic carpets would be "avoid them like the plague," if you will be building a new home.

♪♪♪♪♪

Look no further than the EPA Waterside Mall, headquarters for the Environmental Protection Agency, to learn from the agency's short-sightedness. In the late 1970's, when asked to check the air quality in the office I was visiting, I predicted an epidemic of sick employees in five to ten years. A new carpet seven years later was the final blow to an already poor air quality.

♪♪♪♪♪

Ozonating a carpet can be helpful. However, some new glues that bind synthetic fibers to the backing are so toxic that ozonation can cause serious problems.

Using an air filter may trap significant amount of offgasing particles.[i]

---

[i] Aller-X by Dust Free® 1-800-447-1100.

Old carpets present the problem of mold. Older carpets can be steam-cleaned[i] or covered with a layer of dry baking soda. Allow to stand 24 to 48 hours. Then vacuum. Hotels have accommodated us with one or more of these procedures.

Vents. Mold, dust and all kinds of pollution hide in vents. It is advisable to have them cleaned every year or at least every other year. Be sure that the company does not use any toxic cleaners or oiled brushes.

Not everyone is ready to make drastic changes. With that in mind, we can only recommend you choose less toxic products (like those listed above). By selective and informed purchasing, you will find that your lifestyle does not have to change greatly. It will be well worth your time and effort to reduce the contaminants in your environment.

COMPULSIVE CURES - ANOTHER FORM OF DISASTER

Hasty and compulsive change may cause more stress than the toxins you encounter. Approach changes gradually. As your well-being improves you will be motivated to do more to improve your indoor air quality and take new measures to improve your Accordion Reserve©. Little things mean a lot.

PUBLIC ACCESS -
WORKPLACE, SCHOOLS, PROFESSIONAL OFFICES AND MORE

Many people who take such good care of air quality at home are severely limited in polluted public places, primarily due to poor air quality.

---

[i] Eurosteam National Headquarters: 110 S. Hampton Crowley, TX 76036. 1-800-613-3874. See Appendix D.

Attention to improving air quality by government, employers, public service professionals, health care providers and transportation services can make a big difference:

* Performance and Health Enhancement for the "Healthy:"
Dr. Doris Rapp[5] wrote that children and teachers perform better in a relatively environmentally safe school. Attendance, behavior and scholastic achievement all improved in "safer" schools compared to those built with standard school construction and maintenance. This finding has broad implications for the public at large, since we can all benefit.

* Life-saving for ETI victims:
Improving public access restores their productivity, helps them return from disability status and reduces welfare rosters.

Example "Jennifer" has ETI, but her dentist's office space has many toxins offgasing from equipment, glues, resins and mercury vapor. She is reluctant to go for an appointment and seeks advice on locating an environmentally aware dentist.

Two solutions that would go a long way: introduction of a portable air filtration system – Dust-Free® (above) – or one that also removes mercury.[i]

TROUBLE-MAKERS IN THE HOME

See **Table 16-1** to reference many potential sources that offgas pollutants in the home (and potentially) any environment.

SUMMARY – MAXIMS ON AIR QUALITY

1) Pure air has no odor. Air contains only oxygen, nitrogen and water vapor. A contaminant is any substance added to the above mixture. For all practical purposes, we breathe

---

[i] SMARTAir Solutions. Contact Dr. Donald Robbins. SMARTAir@comcast.net. See Appendix D.

contaminated air. Air is the vehicle for entry of contaminants into your lungs.

2) Depending on your individual susceptibility, contaminated air is possibly toxic, sensitizing, allergy generating or all three. When you breathe air that has an odor, you know for certain that contaminants are present. Many contaminants are non-toxic, but may be scented, such as the fragrance of a rose.

3) Natural scents may still act as sensitizers for susceptible individuals.

4) Many toxic substances (like carbon monoxide and mercury vapor) have no odor.

5) Odors are sometimes introduced into the air as:
   * Camouflage to hide an unpleasant or toxic substance (air freshener).
   * An unpleasant warning that supplements a non-odorous substance (the odor of "natural gas").

7) Each indoor environment has its own array of added chemicals and can cause complaints ranging from mild to severe, from smarting eyes to poor vision, from a stuffy nose to disabling asthma, from a mild circulatory problem to life-threatening cardiovascular disease, from mild mental confusion to serious mental disorders. There is no limit to the symptoms poor air quality can trigger.

8) Improving air quality at home and away is a major factor in restoring Environmental Health. While it is easy to blame government or industry for the pollution problem, taking the first steps at home is a sure way to promote change.

Adhesives
Aerosols
Air deodorizers & sprays
Aluminum pots & pans (heated)
Ammonia
Bleaches
Caulks, glues, sealers
Charcoal – grills & lighter fluid
Chlorinated, fluoridated water
Christmas tree needles – resins
Concrete, leveler
Cosmetics, conditioners, nail polish,
  shampoo
Dentrifices, toothpaste, mouthwash,
  sore throat sprays
Deodorants, anti-perspirants
Detergents, soaps
Disinfectants, oven cleaners
Dyes
Electric blankets (plastic wires)
Exhaust – cars, mowers
Fabrics
Fertilizers, garden products
Flameproof mattresses
Floor cleaners & waxes
Foods, fats & rotted food
Fungicide-treated wallpaper
Gasoline, kerosene, other fuels
Gas stoves & appliances
Hair setting lotions & sprays
Heat-sealed plastic packages
Insecticides, pesticides
Lacquer, mineral spirits, solvents,
  turpentine, varnish
Medications

Mineral oil
Mold
Mothballs & crystals
Mothproofed shelf paper
Newspaper print, inks, solvents
Office products, felt-tip pens, copier
  toner
Oils, lubricants for equipment
Paints, stains, sealants
Paper products
Paraffin & waxes
Permanent press clothing
Pillowcases, sheets (synthetic)
Pine-scented cleaners
Plaster
Plastic casings (computers)
Plastic & vinyl mattress covers,
  shower curtains, tablecloths,
  draperies, wraps & packages
Polishes, waxes, & oils
Preservatives & additives
Refrigerant gas (Freon)
Rubber-backed carpets & pads
Rubbing alcohol
Smoke – burned foods, fireplaces,
  heaters
Sponge rubber
Teflon pots & pans
Tin cans lined with phenol
Tobacco smoke
Vitamins A and E (synthetic)
Wallboard, particle board, plywood,
  veneers, melamine

Table 16.1. Troublemakers in the home (adapted, with permission, from Iris Bell, M.D.)

[1] 1978 Clean Air Task Force on Environmental Cancer, Heart and Lung Diseases.

[2] Pall ML. 2002. NMDA sensitization and stimulation by peroxynitrite, nitric oxide and organic solvents as the mechanism of chemical sensitivity in multiple chemical sensitivity. *FASEB Jl* 16:1407-17.

[3] Golos N, Golbitz FG. 1986. *Coping with Your Allergies.* Simon & Schuster, New York.

[4] www.energytheessenceofenvironmentalhealth.com.

[5] Rapp D. 1996. *Is This Your Child's World?* Bantam Books, New York. 1995. *Environmentally Sick Schools.* Video format. Practical Allergy Relief Foundation, Buffalo, NY.

17
FOOD -
Modifying Your Diet

Prologue

♫♫♫♫♫

My name is Natalie Golos, and I am a "chocoholic." No, I do not know of a Chocoholics Anonymous group, but we could learn a good lesson from Alcoholics Anonymous because Denial is usually the first problem of the food-sensitive and/or allergic individual.

In my earlier books, lectures and group workshops, motivation for diet modification was easy; I was addressing correctly diagnosed patients eager for methods to enjoy food without breaking a very strict diet. Later, I found there is a greater challenge to motivate apparently healthy individuals to practice diet modification. Now that Alan and I have been exploring the ubiquitous virtue of the Accordion Reserve©, we have a pictorial explanation to use for motivating prevention of food addiction.

Before we begin to turn negatives into positives using diet modification, an explanation of food addiction is in order. My most graphic example of food addiction occurred in a maximum-security ward of a private psychiatric institution. I was making rounds with a psychiatrist who wanted my help as he considered preparing a comprehensive environmental control unit to test violent inmates.

One patient had become calm, gentle and pleasant after a five-day water fast that had been recommended by the referring allergist. Because of the patient's previous dietary habits, the allergist had recommended eggs as the first food to be re-

199

introduced. Immediately after eating eggs, the patient became so violent that it took several male attendants to apply restraints necessary to prevent injury to himself and others.

♫♫♫♫

Food-Induced Violence There are countless documented cases of food-induced violence. Is it possible that food allergy and other sensitivities are one of the real explanations for the explosion of violence in our society which indulges itself in junk food, fast food, additive/preservative-filled foods and other poor eating habits? Also, could food allergy be the cause of milder behavioral manifestations involving family squabbles – dissension, teenage rebellion, etc.? For an in-depth study of the problem, read Barbara Reed's book, *Food, Teens & Behavior.*[1]

Food Addiction It usually takes about 96 hours for food to clear the gastrointestinal tract and other parts of the body's food absorption system. With constant repetition your system never becomes free of that food, causing food addiction similar to pharmaceutical drug addiction. Addiction to a drug induces tolerance to it, requiring progressively larger doses to generate an effect.

However, food allergy is more complex because foods are composed of multiple chemicals (some are unidentified) and are altered during their growth, production, maturation, transport and preparation. Foods are further altered during digestion. Distinguishing which substances triggered the food reaction is sometimes confusing and requires professional assessment.

The addiction process called "masking" compounds the problem because you can become a food addict without knowing it.

Masking Suppose you are allergic to corn. If for a period of ten days you avoid eating any form of corn (see also withdrawal below), then reintroduce it into your diet, you are likely to have a definite reaction very quickly or at least within 18 hours. Then, by eating corn every day, your reactions may become weaker and eventually you may not even notice a reaction. You are still allergic to corn but your symptoms are masked (hidden), so you no longer associate the symptoms with the food that caused them.

New symptoms and chronic disorders may develop. Eventually you may feel relief only after eating corn. You then eat corn more and more frequently. Once the problem becomes severe, you begin to crave corn. Corn is the only thing that gives you relief. Corn is your fix!

Food Addiction Cycle Although similar to drug addiction, food presents three additional problems that introduce even more difficulty in diagnosing the underlying cause.

*   Corn oil or corn syrup is found in many prepared foods, making it difficult to know when corn is being introduced into your system.
*   You may be addicted to several foods at once and in varying degrees. This so confuses the issue that only an experienced clinician may be able to decipher the puzzle.
*   Foods are grouped in families according to similar biologic and chemical characteristics. The classifications are hundreds of years old but it was Environmental Medicine pioneers Rinkel, Randolph and Zeller[2] who made the connection between food families and allergies.

Withdrawal While abstaining from a food (or other substance) for hours to several days, withdrawal symptoms may develop. This sequence is called "de-adapting" or "unmasking." In the corn example above, we emphasized the re-exposure that elicited the original symptoms of exposure. As the time increases from the last exposure, symptoms can be identical to, different from or more acute than the original exposure symptoms. It is worth repeating the statement, since it applies equally to withdrawal symptoms: "Substances of exposure are no different from substances of abuse."

Comment The purpose of this chapter is to guide you with diet modification as a starting point. Unless you have already reached rock bottom – critically, chronically and acutely ill, gradually begin to change your eating habits and other substitutions recommended in this book. Diet modification can help prevent food sensitivities or, for those who have mild allergies, help prevent additional trouble. If you or family members have food sensitivities, diet modification allows you to ease into dietary changes.

Don't try to be a one hundred percenter who must do it — all or nothing. When you start to change your diet, make it easier for you and your family by being flexible. As you make changes, use your **Body Awareness** to recognize your increased wellness. The improvement serves as your motivation to take greater steps toward improving your diet.

Linked to our theme of Environmental Health (EH), food allergy prevention is perhaps the easiest and most effective method of building your **Accordion Reserve©**. Changing your eating habits helps counteract unavoidable toxins you encounter.

TRANSITIONAL STEPS FOR ENVIRONMENTAL HEALTH

Begin modifying your eating habits by changing to more wholesome foods:

Sugars Nutrition experts usually recommend cutting back on sugar: honey, maple syrup, grain syrups (corn, rice, molasses, etc.) and especially crystallized beet and cane sugar. Dates, figs, raisins, coconuts and other (unpreserved) dried fruits are better substitutes for sugar; however, if you are yeast or mold sensitive, avoid these also until the problem is resolved or under control.

As you reduce your intake of sweeteners, your need for them will also decrease and you will be able to enjoy the natural sweetness of fresh fruit for snacks and desserts. Be aware that most artificial sweeteners may be toxic to your system and many are considered carcinogenic. Most health food stores carry the white powdered form of stevia, a natural plant that can be used like sugar.

Cooking Cooking is a trade-off. Nutrient quality will be reduced, but certain toxins (from molds or natural toxins) will be inactivated. Unless there is a medical reason for cooking your foods, enjoy the taste and nutrients in raw fruits and vegetables.

Choice of cooking vessels can affect the foods you eat. For example, iron skillets, aluminum pots or Teflon-coated frying pans release molecules when heated and permeate the food.

Junk Food Reduce consumption of junk food. Substitute nuts, sunflower seeds, roasted soybeans and fresh fruit. Buy pure popping corn to make your own wholesome popcorn. If you buy corn chips or potato chips choose brands (preferably organic) which use pure safflower or canola oil, contain no additives or preservatives and are packaged instead of canned. Instead of buying soft drinks and fruit drinks, buy pure fruit juice and natural unflavored sparkling waters (flavor with your own pure fruit juice).

Refined Grains Most nutrients have been removed from refined grains; added to enrich grains, many manufactured nutrients can be harmful. Instead learn to use whole wheat, whole rice and other whole grains.

A note of interest for food-sensitive individuals: Grains are in multiple families – the most familiar family is the grass family. See Appendix A and B for the details.

Salt Because salt places unnecessary stress on your system, become less dependent on it by gradually reducing your consumption. Herbs make a tasty seasoning alternative. However, do not avoid salt if you have a low blood pressure problem related to autonomic nervous system dysfunction. Choose sea salt rather than products that may contain dextrose or phosphates that prevent caking.

Years ago, Chemistry Professor Emeritus from Johns Hopkins University Dr. Alsoph Corwin said that stress from salt could be modified by mixing one part sea salt to one part potassium bicarbonate. He did caution limiting salt if your doctor has recommended a low-salt diet (personal communication to Natalie).

In a Nutshell We have recommended cutting out the worst diet offenders — refined sugars and grains, preservatives (especially nitrates, BHA and BHT) and artificial flavors and colors. Our book places more emphasis on how to change rather than on reasons to change. You can find detailed explanations in Dr. Rapp's book *Is This Your Child?*[3] or Dr. Rea's *Chemical Sensitivities.*[4] Learning more about food sensitivities will help in your commitment to diet modification.

RECOMMENDED CHANGES

Eating Out When changing your dietary habits, you can still eat prudently in restaurants. There are many trade-offs when making choices. An occasional "indiscretion" is not the end of the world, but people who eat many meals in restaurants can choose baked or broiled over fried. Choose a restaurant that will adjust food preparations to your requests. Some restaurants are now advertising at least some foods that are organically prepared. You can also ask your waiter to omit the most tempting breads or rolls before the salad or entrée.

Prepackaged Foods Improve your selections by carefully reading nutrition labels, and whenever possible, omit chemicals, additives and preservatives. Even when the food is pure, packaging may not be. For example, the insides of cans are treated with a sealant.

♫♫♫♫♫

Years ago, before I had a steady supply of organic food, I used to buy frozen vegetables. Although I could tolerate fresh carrots that I prepared, I always reacted to packaged frozen carrots. Dr. Randolph warned me that many frozen foods are packaged in containers that were treated with corn as a preservative. I knew I was sensitive to corn in those days.

♪♪♪♪

Hidden Additives on Labels How often have you reacted to a food although you have read the label very carefully? Be aware of hidden additives not listed on labels. Even new labeling laws do not fully protect you. A label may contain a processed food as an ingredient without labeling the contents of the added processed food. The following are just a few of the many examples of misleading labels:

* *Monosodium Glutamate (MSG)* The Food and Drug Administration (FDA) requires MSG labeling when MSG itself has been added; however, it is possible to find the words "natural flavoring" on labels without any further explanation. That "natural flavoring" could contain MSG. Similarly, it is not necessary to label the MSG that may be found in hydrolyzed yeast. Be very cautious until this misleading label law is resolved.

* *Sulfites* Although the FDA regulates the amount of sulfites in food and requires labeling for them, food may contain hidden sulfites, chemicals known to be fatal to some asthmatics. For example, the label on a processed food might list wine vinegar among the ingredients. However, the label may not tell you that wine vinegar frequently contains sulfites. (See the section in Chapter 19 on "Testing for Food Additives and Pesticides.")

* *Nickel* A different problem in labeling involves terminology. The FDA does not regulate the term "natural" in foods; therefore, it is possible for some manufacturers to label a food "natural" even if it contains hydrogenated oil or margarine processed with nickel used as a catalyst.

DETECTING A FOOD SENSITIVITY

Having been brainwashed to "grin and bear it," we ignore aches and pains, big and small. Or we take an aspirin or other analgesic that temporarily relieves symptoms but does nothing to remove the cause. To determine if a food is causing your symptoms, check out Chapter 19 ("Self-Testing"). In addition, with a little detective work, you can check **Table 19-2**, which was adapted from Dr. Rapp's books (by permission).

MOLD AND YEAST SENSITIVITIES

You are always exposed to mold and yeast. Yeast grows on and within you, just like bacteria and viruses. Most of the time you are able to live comfortably with these organisms present. This is called symbiosis. When your natural protection is altered, growth may not be controlled, which causes symptoms to develop. If you are susceptible, the additional impact of ingested, inhaled or skin-applied molds and yeasts can overload your system.

Medications Over-the-counter or prescription medications may be derived from mold metabolites. Most common are antibiotics and digestive enzymes, which could be aggravating your sensitivities.

Example "Ginny" learned that she was sensitive to mold/yeast in foods. However, she did not connect that the rest of her environment also played a role in her mold sensitivity. When she removed the moldy books from her library (as we discussed in Chapter 16), her symptoms improved.

Molds and yeasts are "cousins" of fungi (members of the same family). If you are sensitive to foods, you should consider cross-reactions to this important group of organisms.

Food Sources for fungi include brewer's and baker's yeasts, mushrooms and the starters for cheeses.

Unexpected Mold Growth on foods adds to the problem. Mold and yeast sensitivities may be especially troublesome for those who live in humid or moldy environments. Poorly functioning refrigerator/freezers accumulate moisture and promote mold growth (as in Chapter 16). Electrical stoppages, accidentally opened doors, poor seals or temperature-recycling failures are causes.

If you have yeast or mold sensitivities, avoid the following foods or use them with caution:

Brewer's Yeast is found in fermented foods, including fruit juices processed in jars or cans, most alcoholic beverages, aged cheeses, soy sauce, cider, sauerkraut and root beer (Dor W. Brown, M.D., personal communication).
Additional sources:
* Vinegar – ingredient in most salad dressings, ketchup, prepared mustard, mayonnaise, pickles, olives, steak sauce and barbecue sauce
* Malt – in many cereals and candies
* Fortified flour, bread and cereal with B vitamins
* Nutritional supplements, unless the label states "yeast free"

Baker's Yeast is found in yeast-leavened breads, rolls and buns, as well as doughnuts, pastries, pizza dough, pretzels and some sourdough products. Some canned refrigerator biscuits and some crackers, cookies, canned soups and flour tortillas also contain baker's yeast.

Mold grows naturally on and in some foods — nuts and seeds, root vegetables, dried fruits, etc. Mold is also airborne. Take certain precautions with foods that contain mold.

By baking nuts or seeds at 325° for 10-15 minutes, you destroy most excess mold, alter or inactivate some mold toxins and release mold-derived chemicals like hexane. Then store them in the freezer to prevent new mold growth and oxidation. In most cases, nut butters prepared from roasted nuts are relatively safe.

Steaming, roasting or broiling can be used for variety. Peeling skins before heating root vegetables can further reduce mold content.

Cheese Depending on your degree of sensitivity, you may be able to tolerate some less moldy cheeses such as cottage cheese, cream cheese, ricotta, mozzarella, Monterey jack and farmer (pot) cheese.

ROTARY DIVERSIFIED DIET

Devised by the late Dr. Herbert J. Rinkel[5] the Rotary Diversified Diet (RDD) is the key to identifying the proper treatment approach for food allergy and sensitivities. Because food addiction is frequently linked to such problems as schizophrenia, alcoholism and obesity, it seems logical that RDD could be used routinely as a first step in the diagnosis and treatment process for these disorders.

RDD is especially appropriate for people who have multiple food sensitivities and can be used as a short-term eating method or for a lifetime. You can use it either to prevent food allergies and addictions or to diagnose and treat food allergies and addictions.

The diet is based on the premise that the most frequently eaten foods are the most common allergens. RDD allows you to eat foods no more than once in four days. Usually four days is needed for food residues to be eliminated from the body.[i]

Food Families Because foods from the same family tend to share common characteristics and often cause similar reactions, you may wish to learn the basics of food families by referring to Appendices A (List I) and B (List II). You can use List II to familiarize yourself with foods and their botanical families (based on biological ori-

---

[i] Bowel transit time is usually 24-48 hours, but food residues may reside in the lining of the gut for 4 days (or more). Therefore RDD is based on the 4-day rule.

gin). To use the alphabetical list (List I), look up the food and note the number shown to the left of that food. Then use that number to refer to List II to locate the appropriate family. Listed under the family name are all closely related foods, botanically or biochemically.

To explore food families in greater depth see *Success in the Clean Bedroom* by Natalie Golos and William Rea.[i] Caution: Severely sensitive individuals should seek professional guidance in using RDD, to recognize, minimize and treat withdrawal reactions.

Ideally, according to Dr. Joseph Morgan, a pediatrician in Coos Bay, Oregon, infancy is the best time to begin rotating foods. Many food allergies may be prevented, as the child learns to eat a large variety of foods without repetition.

In fact, there is now clinical evidence to suggest that allergic parents who eat a rotation diet before conception can, in some cases, prevent food allergies in their unborn child.[ii] Then during pregnancy, the expectant mother can continue rotation to minimize allergy.

Childhood cow's milk allergy may be as frequent as it is because expectant mothers have been encouraged to consume milk daily for its calcium content (and to satisfy that ice cream craving!).

Cravings during pregnancy are an enigma to most of us. Sometimes, this may represent true addiction, food allergies/sensitivities or habit. However, cravings during pregnancy further highlight the complex interaction of hormonal, immune and neurologic factors.

Don't be discouraged by the number of foods you find you cannot tolerate on your RDD. The good news is that later on you will probably be able to tolerate many more foods than in the initial stages of the diet. When you suddenly shift to a rotary diet or have just finished a fast, your system is unusually sensitive and mildly

---

[i] Golos N, Rea W. *Success in the Clean Bedroom.*   Limited supply.   See our website at www.alanrvinitskymd.com.
[ii] Personal communication.

allergenic foods may cause a stronger reaction than normally would be the case. However, foods that caused only minor reactions can be returned to the diet with little or no problem after avoiding them for a few weeks or months.

Cyclic Allergies Many food allergies, called cyclic or non-fixed allergies, come and go depending on frequency of exposure. Non-fixed food allergies may comprise up to 70 to 80 percent of a patient's allergies. With proper management on RDD, some foods that create severe symptoms can later be eaten safely. This happens because the body has had a rest period, during which it regains tolerance. Waiting time varies — some foods can be eaten after a rest period of three to four weeks; for others, it may be necessary to wait two to six months before they can be eaten safely. A few foods may remain permanent allergens.

At times foods may cause mild reactions, and at other times severe, depending on your **Accordion Reserve**©. For example, if you are allergic to trees, and it is tree season, your food allergy to corn may be worse, even when you rotate. If you experience a chemical exposure, such as pesticides, your blueberry allergy may result in eczema or hives. (Organic blueberries may produce no reaction.) If you are sleep-deprived, your sensitivity to apples may be more pronounced.

PRINCIPLES OF THE RDD

Make changes at your own pace, keeping in mind that each change helps increase your **Accordion Reserve**©.

* Eat each food item no more often than once every four days.
* Choose foods with fewer chemical contaminants. Whenever possible, select foods labeled "certified organic." Fresh or frozen foods are better than canned foods.
* Use sea salt for seasoning rather than regular salt, which may contain dextrose, aluminum or other harmful ingredients.

* When dining out, ask questions about food preparation. Choose simple a la carte items, plain meats or fish, fresh fruit and steamed vegetables without sauces.
* Drink and cook with spring water stored and bottled in glass containers.[i]
* Space meals a minimum of three to four hours apart.[ii]
* Eat the desired amount at each meal within one hour. Do not repeat a food in the same day unless directed otherwise.

Nutritional Considerations The nutritional advantages of RDD are many. Because you eat a wide variety of foods, it is easier to achieve a nutritionally balanced diet. Eat whole, unrefined, high-fiber foods. Because these foods have not been processed, they still contain important nutrients. RDD helps ensure that an individual with multiple food omissions still maintains a nutritionally balanced diet. For the very sensitive individual, food choices must be carefully made to ensure adequate caloric, protein, fat, carbohydrate, vitamin and mineral content. Supplements will probably be required, if for no other reason than to accommodate metabolic demands while detoxing. Refer to many published references that list the nutritive content of foods.

Easing into Rotation As stated above, RDD is an involved diet. It can be used to prevent, diagnose or treat food allergies. As a beginning step, this volume introduces the concept of easing gradually into rotating major foods.

FOOD ROTATION MADE EASY

Introduce the idea of rotating foods as a way of educating the family about good eating habits. Involve the whole family in the rotation and not just an allergic individual who would be labeled "sick."

---

[i] Storing filtered tap or well water in non-sterile glass bottles will still encourage mold growth. One of our toddlers became more sensitive to mold after his parents were doing their best to avoid regular tap water.

[ii] Exercise Sandwich® can still be utilized, by eating the same foods before and after the exercise session.

Start rotating animal protein; you can rotate vegetables and fruits later when you are ready. Choosing from the more familiar proteins in Appendix B you could select from the following:

* Day 1 — Monday: Sheep yogurt and sheep feta, lamb or mutton, cod-fish and haddock
* Day 2 — Tuesday: Swordfish or turkey
* Day 3 — Wednesday: Flounder, halibut, sole, goat yogurt and goat milk, ham or pork (uncured)
* Day 4 — Thursday: Sea trout, eggs or chicken

Unless fish is the only animal protein you can eat, eat fish every other day, selecting from the choices given for each day.

Please note that on day 1 and 3 you have meat (lamb, goat or pork), but they are in different families. On day 2 and 4 you have fowl, but they too are in different families. The same is true in the fish families. See Appendix A and B.

After experimenting with animal protein, you may wish to rotate fruit. When rotating fruits or vegetables, you'll have the greatest variety if you wish to split the families, eating members of the same family every other day.

* Day 1 — Monday: Apples
* Day 2 — Tuesday: Oranges
* Day 3 — Wednesday: Pears (same family as apples)
* Day 4 — Thursday: Grapefruit (same family as oranges)

FOODS AND THEIR COMPOSITION

As noted at the outset of this chapter, every food is a complex mixture. Some of the components may be nutritive, toxic or sensitizing. Depending on your individual susceptibility, a component may be perfectly safe, but for someone else, it may prove toxic.

Individual Responses For example, cow's milk may be well tolerated by many individuals. However, an infant with the genetic condition phenylketonuria (PKU) cannot tolerate an amino acid called phenylalanine. If this baby is given a milk-based formula (or even breast-milk), mental retardation will develop.

Fish and the Mercury Problem Caution: Be careful about your choice of fish, shellfish and mollusks. Due to industrial waste and other pollutants, elevated mercury and arsenic content may adversely affect some people who eat fish too often. Whenever possible choose Icelandic and deep saltwater fish, which are apparently less contaminated. Experts have reported that "bottom-feeding fish" are more likely to contain mercury. (Alan says: "Be sure to check their passports!")

Freshwater Fish Industrial and farm runoff carries pesticides, chemical waste and frequently alters water temperature. Animals that feed on freshwater fish are observed to have multiple deformities.[6] You make the decision. We discourage eating freshwater fish.

Other Foods from the Sea Water-sourced foods can also become contaminated by neurotoxins[7] (nervous system poisons). Growing in water where industrial runoff has occurred, algae and other microorganisms emit these neurotoxins. Some fish, shellfish or mollusks may eat this contaminated source, and humans become end-of-the-food-chain recipients.

Fish on the Farm Today you can purchase "farm-raised" fish. It has been reported that the process of "raising" fish results in contamination as well. Like farm-raised grain-fed land animals, grain-fed fish may also have altered essential fatty acid composition.[i]

---

[i] Saltwater fish eat algae, the source of heart-protective omega 3 fats. Grain-fed animals have high omega 6 and low omega 3 fats, which associates with heart disease.

Foods and Other Contaminants Bacteria, viruses, other parasites and organisms and metabolic products (possibly toxic) derived from these sources may contaminate foods.

The Importance of Organic Food

♪♪♪♪♪

Just as you should be aware of the adverse effects of mercury, arsenic, and other neurotoxins, you should likewise be vigilant about chemicals, such as pesticides, preservatives and additives in food. It is rewarding to me to hear conservationists increasingly promoting integrated pest management[i] for lawns, flowers and trees. I hope that soon more emphasis will be placed on the dangers of crops treated with herbicides and pesticides. In addition to the direct toxic effect, the burden of nutrition depletion compounds the effect.

♪♪♪♪♪

Look for code labels on fruits and some vegetables: a five-digit number headed by "9" as in 9xxxx = "organic;" a four-digit number headed by "4" as in 4xxx = "commercial."

When fresh organic produce is not available, you can usually find frozen fruits and vegetables under the label of Cascadian Farms® or Whole Foods Market®. Inquire locally for other sources.

Organic peanut butter, almond butter, cashew butter, tahini (sesame butter) and sunflower butter also can usually be purchased in a health food store. Caution labels have words to the effect: "Made in plants that process peanuts, soy, seeds and tree nuts."

If you are food allergic or gluten-sensitive, you are at risk. An infinitesimal contamination through the atmosphere can affect

---

[i] Integrated pest management is a way of controlling pests in a less toxic manner (to humans, pets, and wildlife). Check with your state or local department of agriculture to learn what is being done to protect us all. See "Beyond Pesticides" in Appendix D.

your rotation. A good Cuisinart will have instructions for homemade nut and seed butters. If your health food store does not carry organic nuts and seeds, buy them through a catalog.

♪♪♪♪♪

Although each of my books about Environmentally Triggered Illness (ETI) has a description of RDD, I continue refining, improving and simplifying the diet. While my books have been well received by physicians and readers, our book, like other diet books, has its limitations. It is impossible to devise a universal diet of any kind, especially an RDD. Just as everyone is unique, so must everyone have a custom-made diet. Diet books can give you only guidelines, whether your goal is to gain or lose weight, maintain a healthy wholesome diet or treat or prevent serious chronic illness (diabetes, heart problems, allergies or ETI, etc).

♪♪♪♪♪

FOOD MORSELS

1) Like air, food is a vehicle for substances to enter the body. Ingested, they enter the body through the gastrointestinal system. Inhaled as molecules (odors), they enter through the nose and lungs.

2) Pure foods provide:
* Calories as proteins, carbohydrates and fats.
* Vitamins and minerals.
* Water.

3) Foods are foreign substances to the body and act as
* Healthy stressors.
* Unhealthy stressors.

4) Reactions to food substances may be allergic, sensitizing or both.

5) Foods can be a source of
* Contaminants.
* Toxins.
* Natural substances that may be toxic or produce undesirable effects in some individuals.

6) Reactions can occur in response to contaminants, natural substances or toxins.

7) Complex reactions may result from the interaction of foods, contaminants and toxins.

8) Regardless of the mechanism of reaction, each event will affect the **Accordion Reserve**[©].

9) Changing your eating habits can help you build your **Accordion Reserve**[©].

10) The RDD is a tool that:
* Aids in the diagnosis of food allergy/sensitivity.
* Promotes a large variety of foods in the diet.
* Aids in the treatment of food allergy/sensitivity.
* Builds the **Accordion Reserve**[©] and balances the autonomic nervous system.

11) Choose foods that are:
* Less contaminated – fewer additives, preservatives, artificial colors and pesticides.
* Less likely to be contaminated – safely handled, packaged and raised; grown organically and less processed.
* Less likely to contribute to the major causes of illness and premature death in our society.

12) Choose to eat in moderation – quantity, quality and diversity.

---

[1] Reed B. 1983. *Food, Teens & Behavior.* Natural Press. Chicago.

[2] Rinkel HJ, Randolph T, Zeller M. 1951. *Food Allergy.* Charles C Thomas, Publisher. Springfield IL.

[3] Rapp D. 1991. *Is This Your Child?* Morrow, New York.

[4] Rea. WJ. 1992-97. *Chemical Sensitivities.* Lewis Press, Boca Raton.

[5] Rinkel HJ. 1936. Food allergy. *J Kansas M Soc* 37:177.

[6] Colborn T, Dumanoski D, Myers JP. 1996. *Our Stolen Future - Are We Threatening Our Fertility, Intelligence, and Survival?: A Scientific Detective Story.* Dutton, New York.

[7] Shoemaker RC. 2001. *Desperation Medicine.* Gateway Press, Inc. Baltimore, MD.

18
WATER -
Protecting Nature's Gift

Prologue

♫♫♫♫

Deserted, Abandoned! Over 150 patients stranded without our allergist who understood Environmentally Triggered Illness (ETI). Due to a family health emergency, Dr. Eloise Kailin moved before she was able to find a doctor to help us.

Because I had already authored my first book, with Dr. Kailin's guidance, the patients turned to me. I was bombarded with calls of desperation from patients whose new doctors insisted: "It's all in your head."

Environmental questions I could answer. Medical questions? I'm not a doctor. Fortunately, I do recognize when it is necessary to send patients back to their referring doctor; back then there were no local Environmental Medicine (EM) doctors. However, we did receive some help thanks to the generosity of leading physicians: the late Dr. Lawrence Dickey, surgeon (former CME Director of AAEM), the late Dr. Theron Randolph, allergist/internist, and my allergist, Dr. Eloise Kailin. When it was necessary, I was given permission to refer local physicians to the appropriate EM — surgeon, internist, allergist.

What Does This Have to Do with Water? Everything! It was the only relatively safe thing I could suggest by myself before hearing from one of the EM physicians. I had been told dehydration is a common problem with ETI patients, frequently a major initial cause or first sign of ETI. Unless a doctor had curtailed consumption of water, I recommended immediately

217

drinking one glass of pure water followed by continuously slowly sipping water until at least 1/2 gallon had been consumed.

♪♪♪♪

LET'S LOOK AT THE BENEFITS

Pure water:
* Helps expand the circulation (as long as adequate salt is present or is consumed simultaneously).
* Flushes the system of toxins that are first processed in the liver. These are rushed to the kidneys and gastrointestinal tract, where they are more effectively cleared from the body when we are well hydrated.
* Calms the emotional system, as a way of distracting negative thoughts.
* Suggesting a visual image of hot water flowing enhances calming by floating away fears and negative thoughts, effecting a gastrointestinal pain catharsis.

♪♪♪♪

The search for pure water reminds me of "Alice." Symptomatic of multiple system illness, Alice had been told by many doctors: "It's all in your head." Alice had spent years and great sums of money going to psychiatrists but with no success. Finally a doctor told her he couldn't help her but suggested she go to Dr. Kailin, an allergist "with some crazy ideas that seem to help some people."

With Dr. Kailin's care, Alice became a functioning, productive leader of a support group. It was she who taught me how to cook exotic foods. After Dr. Kailin's departure, Alice returned to the uninformed doctors. When her digestive system deteriorated, she had trouble with most foods she had previously eaten without reaction.

Symptomatic whenever she drank any form of water, her throat and intestines burned. While I waited for help, I suggested that she try different sources of water. Finally she told her story to a television investigative reporter whom she asked to contact me.

For the TV interview, I selected a few patients who would be demonstrating the wide range of ETI. In contrast to Alice, a septuagenarian, I chose a mother whose 10-month-old was very sensitive to plastic among other things.

The mother described to the reporter how she was treated like an hysterical neurotic. Although she pleaded with hospital staff to refrain from attaching a plastic name tag on her baby's wrist, her requests were ignored. The infant's wrist swelled immediately, and I was called to offer precautions during the child's hospital stay. The mother was then permitted to furnish special bedding and spring water that the baby could tolerate. The staff also arranged for other suggestions I made.

As for Alice, she was <u>flooded</u> with calls from viewers offering samples of well water. She found water she could drink without much difficulty. On my suggestion, she rotated her water, drinking a different source each day of a four-day rotation.

(In addition, during a phone consult with me, Dr. Dickey identified that Alice had hypothyroidism. Dr. Randolph then found a form of thyroid replacement that Alice could tolerate.)

Back to water, so essential to our health, yet so troublesome in its impurities.

"WATER, WATER EVERYWHERE, BUT NOT A DROP TO DRINK"

No, this quotation is not about Samuel Taylor's "Ancient Mariner" sea water. We're discussing polluted waters right here in the United States. In the 60's, Dr. Kailin reported finding

219

detergents in Maryland's Montgomery County wells. In the early 80's water reared its proverbial ugly head during a talk show on my book tour promoting *Coping with Your Allergies.*

A neighboring city's water was so contaminated that water was being shipped in from Binghamton, New York. A caller asked if it were safe to bathe in the water. Not wanting to cause a panic before the evidence was reported, but compelled to offer an honest response, I said it depends on the cause of the contamination. To temper my response, I casually suggested ways to be on the safe side for babies, allergic patients and people with sensitive skin:

* Buy spring water bottled in glass (not plastic).
* Sponge bathe in your drinking water.
* Rinse and cook your food in drinking water.

Later that day, as I was lecturing to a group, I was told that the two cities had the same source of water. Contaminated water was trucked into the area to replace contaminated water!! An isolated case? Were the rumors true? Who knows? With old water pipes and frequent water main breaks, the pounding on those pipes loosens crusted sediments that seep into water supplies.

Closer to Home The above polluted water incident occurred in the early 80's. Similar catastrophes have occurred throughout the U.S. The suburban Washington, D.C. area news media has reported episodic water problems from deteriorating pipes. Look no further. Recall in Chapter 12 my personal water emergency that resulted from a main break.

Please learn from my experience. Check if your house water pipes are at the end of the line, beyond the fire hydrant that is used to flush out contaminants. One inspector suggested that there is no way to clean my pipes without a costly reconstruction by Washington Suburban Sanitary Commission. I received no satisfaction and unfortunately gave up.

As we get ready to go to press, there was yet another water main break near my front yard. The sludge that came into my house overloaded my very expensive, efficient new water filter replacements. Even the plumber couldn't stand the foul odor when he removed them.

Turning Negatives into Positives Although my body is again covered with unsightly, itching, burning, painful sores, I keep thanking God for the help of two excellent doctors, Dr. James Brodsky and Dr. Alan Vinitsky. Their treatments are showing success. I also keep thanking God for my Energy Healing process that helps me <u>dampen</u> my pain so that I may continue to function.

I feel compelled to include the above episode to warn people about dangerous water main breaks – a growing problem in the greater Washington, DC area and elsewhere throughout the United States. It can be <u>liquidated</u> by a community effort.

♪♪♪♪

PURE WATER

Water technically contains molecules of H_2O – pure and simple.

CONTAMINATED WATER

An Environmental Protection Agency (EPA) internal study recently "...showed that some companies and municipalities have illegally discharged toxic chemicals or biological waste into waterways for years without government sanctions. Such discharges can cripple fisheries, taint fishing holes and increase the risks of illnesses ranging from skin rash to lead and mercury poisoning."[1]

From the above you can plainly see that any substance, organism or parasite that is dissolved in or lives in pure water is a contaminant. Not every contaminant is toxic, poisonous, infectious or dangerous. For example, minerals dissolved in water obtained from a natural spring may actually be therapeutic.

Considering whether a contaminant is safe may become a costly commercial adventure. In Chapter 19: "Self Testing" you may be able to discover some hints to help you decide if more thorough testing is required. On the other hand, if you clearly have symptoms that seem to be related to drinking water, a personal medical evaluation may be required to determine if you harbor a parasite like giardia.

During your testing, you may need to obtain a glass-bottled water source. Most of our patients use Mountain Valley® Spring water, the one most frequently tolerated by ETI patients. Yet it does contain mineral content and some contaminants.[i]

Water Filters A filtration system should be used to rid water of its toxic, poisonous or dangerous qualities. Given the broad selection of water filters – some quite expensive, how do you find a functional system, and at what cost? First consider your budget.

Systems Options You can install filters at each sink for drinking, at tubs/showers for bathing, at toilets and at washing machines. Or you can install a whole-house system at the water inlet. Filtration units include a variety of charcoal, ceramic or mixed cartridges and reverse osmosis units, alone or in series. There are even water purification systems with water-energizing features. Your own home requirements usually depend on the composition of the water source that supplies your house. Therefore, if it is financially feasible, or if you suspect a contaminant problem that is specifically affecting your health, test your water.[ii]

---

[i] Despite its fine reputation, Mountain Valley® has started to market water in plastic containers in some areas. No doubt this decision is a result of financial and convenience pressure. For example, at a swimming pool or during exercise, it may not be practical to carry glass. Yet, at home, where choice is available, clearly glass bottles are preferable.

[ii] Reputations are important to rely on. As always, careful choices depend on price, quality and availability.

You can even choose to be redundant — whole-house filtration and a second filter at a drinking or showering site, depending on individual sensitivities. Also available are units for treating pool water.

Remember: Water filtered at the house inlet flows through pipes of copper, (lead), PVC and other materials. Even a redundant system may not get all of the lead out, because the spigot is in line after the last filter.

Filtration is recommended for removing:
* Volatilized and aerosolized chlorine and "halogenated organic matter" (think "chloroform-like") in city chlorine-treated water. Chlorine aerosolizes when toilets are flushed and hot showers taken, resulting in contamination of indoor air quality.
* Trace amounts of chemicals, excess minerals, toxic metals and organisms (parasites, bacteria, viruses).

Distilled Water Some experts recommend distilled water as the safest form of pure water. Theoretically all impurities and contaminants have been removed. That depends on the equipment used and the source of the water prior to distillation. Some contaminants have the same boiling point as water; therefore, the fraction distilling at the same time would contaminant the distilled water.

We make these additional observations about distilled water:
* We know of no companies that dispense distilled water in glass.
* Purity and distillation equipment should be made of glass or stainless steel.
* Seals or fittings of distillation equipment may trap contaminants and release them during subsequent distillations.
* Home distillers transfer contaminants in the water to the air where the equipment functions.

SUMMARY

*   Whatever your source, it is best to use water from glass containers, when the water is bottled at the source. Home filling of bottles with tap or other water can become a source of mold.

*   Use your drinking water for cooking and medical purposes – such as taking enemas and cleansing your sinuses with the Neti Pot (See Chapter 12).

*   Water is so vital to your health that using pure water is a life-giving, **Accordion Reserve**©-expanding force.

---

[1] Gugliotta G, Pianin E. "EPA: Few Fined for Polluting Water. Agency Says It Must Do Better Job of Monitoring." *The Washington Post*, June 6, 2003.

19

SELF-TESTING –
Product (In)Tolerance
Labels and Advertising "Show and Tell"

Prologue

Fateful Harvest You have to test before buying anything. Don't take our word for it. By permission, we present excerpts from the book jacket and from a few pages of *Fateful Harvest.*[i]

"Duff Wilson is a reporter at the Seattle Times. His work has been awarded a Goldsmith Prize for Investigative Reporting from Harvard University and was a finalist for the Pulitzer Prize for Public Service." (Book jacket)

Mr. Wilson wrote: "…Chemical manufacturers are disposing of leftover toxic waste by selling it to unsuspecting farmers as fertilizer. The tainted fertilizer – containing arsenic and cadmium, lead and dioxins – is believed to be destroying crops, sickening animals, and endangering the nation's food supply. And owing to a gaping regulatory loophole, it is completely legal.

"Fertilizer companies sold recycled toxic waste in blended products for backyard gardeners and golf course owners, too. Toxicologists told me traces of poison in the retail fertilizer market would be more dangerous than in farm products because homeowners lay it on so thick and leave it out where the kids and pets can touch it.

---

[i] Wilson D. 2001. *Fateful Harvest.* Harper Collins, NY. We recommend that you take a copy of *Fateful Harvest* to lawn care companies, landscape designers, garden clubs, and anyone who does gardening.

"There were, of course, no warning labels. There were no limits. And I could not find a single government agency in America that had analyzed fertilizer for the unadvertised ingredients. So I did it myself.

"I bought twenty common products at home and garden stores and delivered them, unopened, to an accredited laboratory a few blocks from the Seattle Times. Frontier Geosciences analyzed fourteen toxic metals.

"One of those was a white plastic jar decorated with a drawing of a garden. I bought it at the True Value hardware down the street from my home. The label said: 'NuLife All Purpose Trace Elements is a mixture of the most common elements.'

"I asked the clerk what it was. She squinted at the fine print and said, 'It's like an expensive multivitamin.'

"I came to treasure that cup-sized jar. NuLife All Purpose Trace Elements was nothing more or less than a highly toxic hazardous waste captured from the pollution control device of a steel smelter, wetted with acid and rolled into dark brown granules to look like fertilizer, and sold in my neighborhood hardware store. It even smelled of metal.

"I learned a smelter somewhere paid $100 to $200 a ton to get rid of the toxic waste I was holding. I paid $4.49, plus tax, for twelve ounces. No wonder, as I walked out of the hardware store, I had a spooky feeling that I was part of a vast, unknowing network of people helping heavy industry save money by sprinkling its hazardous wastes on our land."

♪♪♪♪

Years ago when asked to testify at the Toxic Substance Control Act Hearing, I recommended that tests of toxic substances be performed on humans before introducing them in the marketplace.

When challenged that human tests were dangerous and against the law, I replied: "Isn't that what industry is continuously doing? Every time consumers purchase a product they are testing it. Unfortunately, some of the most toxic products have been labeled safe until proven dangerous. The solution is to use an environmentally controlled unit to test people before placing any product on the market."

A disturbing example occurred in the government-required vaccine program. In hindsight, a preservative containing mercury[i] has been removed from most children's vaccines, as a precautionary measure because the cumulative dose exceeded federal guidelines for possible toxicity. Why was the vaccine industry permitted to use it for so long?[ii, iii]

♪♪♪♪♪

Many other examples come to mind – chlorinated pesticides, organophosphate pesticides, calcium cyclamate (an artificial sweetener), diethylstilbestrol, thalidomide and many more.

Case in Point When first introduced, polyester was considered a miracle fabric, relegating cotton to an undesirable status. As demand decreased, American cotton was exported. Then it happened. People in droves rejected polyester – some people recognized symptoms; others felt uncomfortable but did not know why (thus the need for testing).

To recoup their losses, manufacturers saved the polyester industry by making blends, thus reducing obvious symptoms and dis-

---

[i] Thimerosal. *Immunization Saftey Review: Vaccines and Autism.* 2004 (in press). National Academies Press, Washington.

[ii] House Committee on Government Hearing, November 14, 2002, Chairman Honorable Dan Burton, Re: Mercury and Dental Amalgams and Vaccines: An Examination of the Science.

[iii] National Vaccine Information Center. See Appendix D.

comfort. Madison Avenue took charge with an effective advertising campaign. It's not what they said, but what they didn't say. So except for the most sensitive patients, people began using blends, not obviously reacting, but reducing their Accordion Reserve[©].

♫♫♫♫♫

Even labeling laws do not protect people. Years ago when I was in Texas to help Dr. Rea in his Environmental Control Unit, the nurses asked me why patients could sometimes tolerate and sometimes react to cotton towels. As I checked the linen closets, I found all towels were labeled 100% cotton. However, the back label on some towels indicated a percentage of polyester was woven into interfacing or trimming. These very sensitive patients could detect that relatively small amount of polyester.

If you are among the "healthy" and you have some unexplained symptoms, you might consider the possibility that your clothing could be a trigger.

♫♫♫♫♫

Denial How often have you heard someone say, "I am perfectly healthy. I have no allergies and chemicals do not bother me. I am not affected by pollution." Later in conversation, the same individual will make a statement like, "Oh, I can't stand her perfume!" or "Isn't that man's cigar awful?" or "Radishes repeat on me." An acquaintance named "Crystal" once said, "I'm not allergic to smoke. It's just that if there are too many people smoking, my eyes begin to burn. But that can happen to anyone."

As the Accordion Reserve[©] illustrates, the whole point is that it can happen to anyone. Some toxins and foods cause minor reactions. To people with Environmentally Triggered Illness, the reactions are more pronounced, and in some cases totally incapacitating. (Technically, Crystal's symptoms could be allergy-, irritant-, or sensitivity-induced. It's not the mechanism that counts here, but the discomforting effect on the Accordion Reserve[©].)

228

And what does this have to do with self-testing? Everyone can benefit. With no experience and a little knowledge, you save money as you safeguard your health from unwise purchases or belongings that can easily and inexpensively be replaced. There are many different tests that you can use depending on your need from one extreme to the other: for prevention or for disabling chronic illness.

♪♪♪♪

There is a simple test that can be used universally: I used it in its variations during my most critical period and continue to do so today with every purchase where it is applicable.

♪♪♪♪

TESTING FOR CONTAMINANTS IN YOUR AIR SPACE

Sniff Test Testing is best performed in a clean air environment. That is most likely at home, where you have more control. Testing is useful when you are reasonably certain that the substance to be evaluated is a nuisance, but not life-threatening. Detailed monitoring requires some planning, equipment, your personal grounding and **Body Awareness**, and recording your observed symptoms and signs during and after sniff test challenge. **Taking time to monitor yourself tunes you in to your Autonomic Nervous System responses.** The test has several variations:

If you suspect you are susceptible to a toxin in a particular product, avoid that product for two or three weeks and then test it. Frequently the test is valid even when avoidance is not possible.

* *Glass Jar Contaminant Concentrator* Place a sample of fabric or other material in a glass jar (at least quart-size), and close the lid tightly for 36 to 48 hours.
* *Body Proximity Challenge* Place material close to your face/nose in an out-of-the-house setting.

229

An out-of-the-home setting requires that you tune in to your **Body Awareness** and that you detect changes from the way you feel immediately before the test challenge.

Sniff When Ready First thing in the morning before eating or after a walk in fresh air, open the jar for the first time after it has stored the test item, and hold the jar close to your nose, breathing normally for 10 to 15 minutes. If you do not use the glass jar to concentrate any off-gasing fumes, place the material close to your face and nose, breathing normally, as above.

If your testing is not conclusive, you may wish to use a more definitive procedure. Don't try to be a "100 percenter." Use as much of the procedures below as you need. Just don't be compulsive about the procedure. The stress of compulsive action can influence the outcome of your testing.

EQUIPMENT FOR COMPREHENSIVE TEST

* Watch with a second hand (to check pulse)
* Pencil and 3x5 index cards (4 for each test) to record observations
* Mirror (to check changes in face and eyes)
* An observer, when possible, to check things you fail to notice, like being fidgety, scratching and other behavioral manifestations
* Blood pressure monitor (especially for individuals with "labile" or "white coat" hypertension)
* Quart or half-gallon Mason canning jar (to enclose the test sample) where applicable
* Peak flow meter for asthmatics (This instrument and other similar ones can be very useful in detecting asthmatic reactions. In *Is This Your Child?*[1] Doris Rapp gives a detailed explanation of the use of the peak flow meter.)

Testing Time If possible, test during a vacation or weekend, when you are relaxed and not under pressure. As you proceed, testing becomes so automatic that you will recognize positive reactions almost immediately, making the rest of the procedure unnecessary.

TESTING PROCEDURE

Baselines Vital signs (blood pressure, pulse, temperature and respirations) and other personal signs/symptoms are useful information before you begin your testing. This will give you a baseline for comparison during the test.

♫♫♫♫♫

Before treating any autonomic neuropathy in my office, I hand out a diary sheet, requesting baseline measurements of blood pressure and pulse 3 times daily – on arising, mid-day and mid-evening. Usually sympathetic nervous system activity is at its peak from 6 am until noon, so your baseline measurements will vary at different times of the day.

Other observations could include:
* *what symptoms you have:*
  * *example: mucus production, when you have it, where you are when it occurs, anything that relieves it and so on.*

I always tell my patients that they are always acting as my eyes, ears and hands, when I am not with them. In fact, I am a much better diagnostician when they are a major contributor to the discovery process.
♫♫♫♫♫

Finding Your Pulse (for Beginners) If you are using your left wrist to take a pulse, place the tips of your right index and middle fingers on the thumb side of the inside of the wrist about one inch above the hand. You have located the pulse when you feel a throbbing. You can also find a pulse on the side of your neck under the jawbone, about halfway between the chin and the ear.

231

PROCEDURE

* Before beginning any test, practice SHORTCUT to Meditation/Relaxation breathing three times.
* Check your temperature 5 minutes before and 20 minutes after each test, and your pulse 5 minutes before and 10, 20, 40 and 60 minutes after each test.
* A temperature change that cannot be attributed to anything else usually indicates a reaction.
* A pulse increase or decrease of 20 or more beats per minute also usually indicates a reaction.
* Blood pressure (in susceptible individuals) typically increases as well. Occasionally blood pressure may drop.
* Be sure to check your pulse for a full 60 seconds for a true reading; sometimes the rate speeds up or slows down sporadically.
* A DIARY may help you discover a pattern. At the top of each page copy the following chart (**Figure 19-1**). Start a new test on a new page. You may need several pages for a test.

Date & Time	Food	Chemical Stress	Interpersonal Stress	Symptoms	Measures to Relieve Symptoms	Comments

Figure 19-1. Diary headings for charting symptoms related to foods or other stresses.

Use the above chart describing how to record all symptom changes, even if they are as simple as a slight headache, backache or cough; a few sneezes; or a cramp in your toe or foot. Measure and record your pulse and blood pressure in the Symptoms column.

As stated before, the best time to test anything — whatever it may be — is first thing in the morning after taking your pulse and temperature. You can also improve the likelihood of detecting a reaction by walking briskly (minimum of 10 minutes) when the air quality is in the "good" range, and performing the test immediately after you return. Record under Food, or if testing a product, record it under Chemical Stress. Add any stress (exposure) even if you are not testing it.

If your test is inconclusive, repeat it some other day, keeping track as much as possible of things you do that day, foods you eat, and your activities, even if they are as routine as going to the office, driving your car, stopping for gas, shopping or whatever. Record any change in symptoms.

Physical Changes In addition to pulse and blood pressure, look for any change in your appearance, especially color in your hands and face, skin, fingernails and whites of your eyes.

Check your handwriting to test your coordination. Before testing and 5 minutes, 30 minutes and 6 hours after the test, write the same piece of information (your name and full address for example) four different times on four index cards, one for each observation period. Label each card (time and circumstances, e.g. before exposure, 5 min, 30 min or 6 hr, and the substance being tested). (Compare them only after you have completed writing all four cards.) Deteriorating penmanship may indicate that the item being tested affects your coordination.

Observation If possible have someone else observe you while you are testing; another person may observe things you fail to notice, such as scratching, restlessness or other behavioral manifestations.

Spacing Your Tests Wait 3 days between chemical tests. Certain substances may cause delayed reactions. Waiting 3 days between chemical tests makes it easier to detect which irritant is causing your problem. If you are unsure of the results of a test, wait 2 weeks before testing that item again.

You can test foods more frequently. Although people may not react to a chemical for at least 72 hours after exposure, even a person who is a delayed reactor will usually react to a food more quickly. With a food, it has been observed that 90% will react within 4 hours, 9% with a weak but immediate reaction and a stronger one later and 1% delayed over 12 hours but within 18 hours. Skin reactions like itching may occur quickly, but a rash may take a day to develop.

If severe reactions continue for any length of time, it is wise to suspend testing until they clear up unless, of course, they are symptoms that you recognize as having started before your testing began. You must define each individual reaction: how long it takes and when it terminates. Otherwise, confusion will occur.

If you have chronic symptoms that have nothing to do with testing and you cannot go to a doctor's office immediately, delay testing until you can schedule either a visit or a phone consultation with your health care provider. Forwarding your diaries to your practitioner may aide him in discovering responses that you had not noticed.

Food Testing

Food sensitivity can sometimes be detected very easily with a simple food test; at other times it can be so complicated that it requires controlled supervision.

An example of a very serious problem with a very simple solution is the case of an eight-year-old girl with chronic bed-wetting. Her parents did everything possible, including waking her up several times during the night, but she continued to wet the bed. A medical friend of the family suggested eliminating citrus fruit from the child's diet. As soon as the citrus was eliminated, the girl stopped wetting the bed. When the child again ate citrus fruit, as a test, she wet the bed again.

Note: Bed-wetting has many causes and triggers. Citrus juice exposure can trigger bed-wetting or other symptoms, just as any other substance can do. Food testing is helpful but is not precise. It points you in a direction that needs confirmation.

Knowledge of Food Sensitivities Before you do any type of testing for foods, even a simple one-food elimination test, it is important to understand hidden food sensitivities, food families and the rotation diet. So carefully recheck Chapter 17: "Food – Modifying Your Diet." Afterward, you may be able to do a simple food-elimination test.

Suspect foods are those that
* You eat daily.
* You crave.
* **Eliminate** your discomfort right after eating.
* **Cause** discomfort immediately after eating (cough, headache or other symptoms).

Simple Food Elimination Use the section labeled <u>PROCE-DURE</u> and <u>DIARY</u> (**Figure 19-1**), both described earlier in this chapter.

For a challenge food test to be valid, you must avoid the food long enough for possible symptoms to show up, but not so long that you can readapt to the food. The average time for unmasking is 4 days; some people can readapt within 12 days. Although you can perform valid testing by avoiding the food for 5 to 11 days, we suggest you stay on the safe side and avoid the food and members of that food family for 7 to 10 days.

When the avoidance period is over, eat about half a cup of the food before eating anything else that day. Wait an hour. If discomfort occurs immediately, you are likely sensitive to that food. If there is no immediate reaction or symptoms are minor, and you want to check it thoroughly, eat as much of that food as possible that day. If you experience behavior changes or other problems within 18 hours of the time you stop eating this food, you will know that you are probably allergic to that food. Sometimes other allergies that you don't know about can confuse the picture and make the test inconclusive.

If you discover a food allergy, try to avoid the offender and related foods for three to six months. In that time, you may regain a tolerance for it. If so, eat the food no more than once every fifth day so you do not reactivate the allergy.

If you suspect that too many foods are distressing you, you must seek professional medical care. Remember – severe food restrictions may pose more trouble than the original food itself.

Trial Elimination Diet If you suspect that there are many foods involved, a faster way to test them is by eliminating certain groups of foods from your diet for eight days. To do this you must understand the information outlined in the section on food families. It is best not to eat prepared foods during this period because hidden ingredients could throw your test results off. We recommend that you eat only foods cooked from scratch.

Totally eliminate eight groups of food – the eight groups of foods that generally cause the greatest amount of difficulty (see **Table 19-1**). Even a crumb of one of these foods, such as corn, can throw off the test. In addition, if you know of one or two foods that cause you serious reactions, eliminate those, too. During the eight-day period, concentrate on eating a lot of fruits, vegetables and animal proteins other than those on the elimination list.

ELIMINATION DIET

Multiple Food Elimination Test Follow instructions and procedures for testing in the same way that you did for the simple elimination test. During the 8 days of food elimination and the subsequent food testing, carefully keep your diary as did before. Use as many pages per day as needed. Begin testing on the 9th day.

You may discover the following pattern during your 8 days of elimination. The first 4 days may be uncomfortable because of withdrawal symptoms. The next four days may show dramatic improvement and are a reminder that you are on the right track. As yet you don't know which foods are the culprits just that probably some foods are.

Elimination List See **Table 19-1** to eliminate all of the following groups of foods from your diet for eight days:

Group 1	Wheat and all wheat products
Group 2	Chicken, eggs
Group 3	Corn and all corn products, including corn syrup
Group 4	Beef and dairy products, including milk, cheese, whey, nonfat dry milk solids and calcium caseinate
Group 5	Cane sugar, beet sugar and molasses
Group 6	Soy and all soy products, including tofu
Group 7	Coffee, tea and cocoa
Group 8	Peanuts

Table 19-1. Food Elimination List.

The first day of testing, test only group one, which includes wheat and all wheat products. Follow the procedure outlined in the simple food elimination. On day two test group two, chicken eggs, and continue in this manner for the eight days. If you have multiple food and chemical sensitivities, there may be very little change in your symptom pattern. In that case it would be wise to seek the help of a health provider knowledgeable in food allergies (see Appendix D, "American Academy of Environmental Medicine").

After You Test a Food Group As an example, you are fairly certain that Group 1 foods (wheat products) are not your problem. You tested this group on day 9. We recommend that you reintroduce wheat products on day 13 and every 4 days thereafter. This suggestion is based on the principle of the Rotation described in Chapter 17. This sample principle for reintroducing foods can be applied during testing of each additional group. If you think the group may have caused problems, do not reintroduce it during the remainder of the testing, because those foods would likely confuse the remainder of the tests.

Recall the citrus/bed-wetting connection. Not every trigger causes every symptom or condition. Not every condition is caused by every trigger. **Table 19-2**[2] offers clues for consideration. In other words, the table provides possible answers to the following question:

I have <u>symptom (condition)</u>. What trigger could be causing it?

Scan **Table 19-2** to see if any listed problem applies to you with the following limitations. As an example, look at "HIVES." All listed foods or substances do not cause hives in everybody, and there may be foods or substances that are not listed which can **ALSO** cause hives.

Example: One man experienced hives for 10 years. None of the foods caused him any difficulty. During the course of history taking, he revealed that 10 years prior his wife had changed bedding from pure cotton sheets and pillow cases to no-iron polyester. When he returned to cotton bedding, the hives disappeared.

As you scan the chart, make a note of chemicals as well as food.

TESTING FOR FOOD ADDITIVES AND PESTICIDES

If you reacted to food groups in your testing above, the actual food may not be the cause of your symptoms. Food additives, pesticides or even mold could be the culprit:

* Molds grow on dried fruit, nuts, fresh fruits and vegetables. Sooner or later molds grow on everything.
* Sulfur dioxide – A preservative used in treating dried fruit. If labeling is not available, color of the fruit may offer a clue. Brown apricots are naturally dried; yellow apricots are treated.
* Sulfites – A preservative in wines (and possibly at salad bars). A product label may indicate "wine" as an ingredient, but not mention that the wine had sulfites in it.

MEDICAL PROBLEMS AND POSSIBLE MAJOR FOOD OR OTHER SUSPECTS	
ARTHRITIS OR JOINT TIGHTNESS:	Potato*, Tomato*, Green & Red Pepper*, Pimento*, Eggplant*, Chili Pepper* Tobacco*, Wheat or Grains, Milk, Sugar, Beef, Pork, Ham, Bacon, Lard, Chicken, Egg, Coffee, Tea, Food Coloring, Mold, Chemicals, Natural Gas, Gasoline (*Avoid nightshades for 6-9 months to see if these are factors.)
BAD BREATH:	Milk, Wheat, Egg, Yeast or Candida Infections
BED-WETTING:	Milk, Fruit Juices — Orange, Apple, Grape, Grapefruit, Pineapple; Egg, Wheat, Pork, Tomato, Chicken, Cola, Cocoa, Onion, Fish, Cinnamon, Apple, Peanut, Corn, Preservatives, Artificial Colors
COLITIS:	Milk, Wheat, Egg, Corn, Cocoa, Nuts, Orange, Pork, Beef, Chicken, Peanut, Sugar, Tomatoes, Mold, Yeast
CONVULSIONS:	Milk, Egg, Yeast, Mold, Chicken, any food, Vitamin B (derived from yeast)
CYSTITIS:	Tea, Milk (Cheese), Orange or Other Fruit Juices, Sugar, Preservatives, Grape, Coffee, Cola, Corn, Nuts, Dust, Pollen, Mold, Natural Gas, Exhaust Fumes
EAR PROBLEMS:	Milk, Egg, Chocolate, Peanut, Corn, Chicken, Wheat, Dust, Pets, Mold
ECZEMA:	Milk, Egg, Chocolate, Nuts, Potato, Peanut, Peanut Butter, Grains, Yeast, Dust, Pollen, Mold (**Itching and redness when the food is eaten. Skin rash appears the next day.**)
GALL BLADDER DISEASE:	Chocolate, Egg, Pork, Onion, Chicken, Milk, Coffee, Orange, Corn, Bean, Nuts
HEADACHE:	Milk, Chocolate, Cheese, Chicken, Coffee, Shrimp, Egg, Corn, Peanut, Pea, Bean, Cinnamon, Pork, Garlic, Food Coloring, Red Wine, Pollen, Mold, Dust, Pets, Air Pollution, Auto Exhaust, Tobacco Smoke, Paint Fumes, Perfumes, Chemical Odors, Natural Gas
HIGH BLOOD PRESSSURE:	Coffee, Chocolate, Corn, Nuts, Pork, Peanut, Peanut Butter, Milk, Wheat, Rice, Beef, Shrimp, Seafood, Chicken (Add measurement of blood pressure to testing parameters.)
HIVES:	Chocolate, Milk, Egg, Peanut, Cinnamon, Shellfish, Celery, Nuts, Preservatives, Artificial Coloring or Flavors, Spices, Aspirin, Penicillin, "Any" Antibiotic or Drug (**It's what happened before the first hive or next severe outbreak that counts.**)

Table 19-2. Medical Problems and Possible Major Food or Other Suspects.

MEDICAL PROBLEMS AND POSSIBLE MAJOR FOOD OR OTHER SUSPECTS

HYPERACTIVITY:	Artificial Colors (especially Red and Yellow), Sugar (Cane or Beet), Milk, Corn, Cocoa, Wheat, Egg; Apple, Grape (and their Juices); Peanut, Peanut Butter, Tomato, Preservatives, Artificial Flavors, Banana, Orange, Yeast, Dust, Mold, Pollen, Chemical Odors
INFECTIONS:	Milk, Egg, Corn, Wheat, Cinnamon, Spices, Citrus (Orange, Lemon, Lime, Grapefruit), Chocolate, Cola, Mold, Dust
Ear Infections:	Natural Gas, Milk (see also **Ear Problems** above)
Colds:	Egg, Corn, Wheat
KIDNEY PROBLEMS:	Milk, Wheat, Citrus, Grass
MUSCLE PAIN:	Wheat or Grains, Chocolate, Citrus, Corn, Milk, Mold, Chemical Odors, *Synthetic* Carpet
NOSE PROBLEMS:	Milk, Chocolate, Egg, Wheat, Artificial Colors, Yeast, Dust, Pollen, Mold, Pets
OBESITY:	Dairy — Cheese, Milk, Yogurt, Ice Cream; Wheat or Baked Goods, Sugar, Chocolate
SEASONAL HIVES:	Strawberry, Melon, Tomato
SUDDEN SLEEPINESS WHILE EATING:	Beef
ULCER (DUODENAL):	Especially Milk; Also Chicken, Wheat, Corn, Egg, Beef, Tomato, Coffee, Tea, Orange, Avocado, Peach, Potato, Barley, Chocolate, Grape, Peanut, Peanut Butter, Spices
ULCERS IN MOUTH:	Citrus, Vitamin C, Pickles, Apple, Vinegar, Coffee, Chocolate, Potato, Nuts, Cinnamon, Mint, Mouthwash, Mouth Fresheners, Toothpaste
WEAK LEGS:	Grains, especially Wheat; Orange, Mold, Candida
WHEEZING & ASTHMA:	Milk, Egg, Wheat or any Grain, Fish, Shellfish, Peanut, Peanut Butter, Cocoa, Corn, Nuts, Onion, Garlic, Yeast, Cat, Dog, Dust, Pollen, Mold, Aspirin, Tartrazine Yellow Dyes, Sulfites, Perfume, Chemical Odors, Auto Exhaust, Tobacco Smoke

Table 19-2 (continued). Medical Problems and Possible Major Food or Other Suspects. Symptoms may be caused by many different exposures. Not every symptom is triggered by every substance listed.

Most food additives are synthetic chemicals, which may trigger delayed reactions after 3 to 5 days!

To avoid confusion, test foods that are organically grown, unseasoned, and baked or steamed.

Confounding Variables in Testing Sometimes when you test for food sensitivities, your results may be confusing or misleading. Recall that foods are complex mixtures of chemicals, some of which may produce symptoms that are non-immunologic. For example, the nightshades contain chemicals that mimic some pesticide action. Cabbage, broccoli, brussels sprouts, cauliflower, sweet potato and legumes contain natural chemicals that can cause goiter and neuropathy. Bananas and cheese have amines that raise blood pressure. Some foods release histamines — egg white, shellfish, strawberry, tomato, fish, pork and chocolate. Other foods have toxins from mold, algae, parasites and fish.

Persistent health problems during the test indicate that you may be reacting to some other substance. Removing one irritant may not be enough to show a noticeable improvement. Any condition may be caused by something other than food sensitivities and should be checked by a practitioner. But even a minor improvement in well-being indicates the benefit of pursuing testing and using preventive measures.

You can read about more comprehensive testing in *Success in the Clean Bedroom.*[i]

SUMMARY –
TESTING BODY AWARENESS CONNECTIONS

Trust your instincts. Listen to (and observe) what your body is telling you — how your autonomic nervous system responds to

---

[i] Golos N, Rea WJ. 1992. *Success in the Clean Bedroom*. Pinnacle, Rochester. Limited supply. See www.alanvinitskymd.com for details.

your interactions with your environment and your energy. You are playing your Accordion with every test you perform.

With practice you will come to value testing, as Natalie has. Almost certainly you will establish the following connections:

* You can be your best detective.
* You can be your best advocate.
* You are practicing Dr. Randolph's discoveries:
  * Listening, observing and connecting your patterns with a trigger.
  * Learning that symptom suppression with medications is not a substitute for healing.
* In a relaxed state:
  * Sense the variations in your vibrations that help you pinpoint what part of your body is reacting to a trigger (biological, chemical or physical).
  * With practice, you can begin to reduce reactions, thereby initiating your personal **Energy Healing**.

---

[1] Rapp D. 1991. *Is This Your Child?* William Morrow & Co., New York.
[2] Rapp D. 1979. *Allergies and the Hyperactive Child.* Sovereign Books, New York. Adapted with permission.

PART VII

Positive Mental Attitude

CLIMAX

20

CLEANSING YOUR SOUL -
"The Truth Shall Make You Free."
— John 8:32[1]

Prologue

In what follows, "soul" refers to that aspect of a person which is in contrast to the body, mind and spirit. We see soul as the seat of will. Your soul makes the choice to pursue physical, materialistic and self-centered goals or spiritual goals of health as wholeness, spiritual oneness plus love of God and neighbor. To say this another way, your soul is the interface between your body or "false ego" and your spiritual dimension. For most religious traditions, it is the soul that transcends death.

Soul cleansing is neither new nor strange. You have been soul cleansing all your life. Spontaneous reminiscing, when negative, is your body's way of armoring; when positive, it's nature's way of soul cleansing. Dreams are examples of nature's positive soul cleansing. In addition, you can develop positive procedures for processing traumas in a healthy, grounded, relaxed way, which is a concept of the Accordion Reserve©.

MIND, BODY, SOUL, SPIRIT

Throughout our book you have read about Mind/body/soul/spirit. What happens when there is a disconnect among its parts?

In fact, you can observe that each component is unique but is not able to stand on its own. Each component is interdependent and, when united, is greater than the sum of its parts.

Use the following symbols to understand the above concept:
*   — represents separation or disconnect
*   / represents bonding or uniting
*   The capital letter of each component symbolizes its in-dependence

Some of the combinations are:
*   Mind—Body—Soul—Spirit means total disconnect
*   mind/body—Soul—Spirit means disconnect from your soul and spirit
*   Mind—body/soul—Spirit
*   Mind—Body—soul/spirit
*   mind/body/soul—Spirit
*   mind/body—soul/spirit
*   Mind—body/soul/spirit
*   Mind/body/soul/spirit means the Accordion Reserve© at your most powerful Spiritual Healing

♫♫♫♫♫

Spontaneous Cleansing Beautiful music, art and nature frequently evoke spontaneous soul cleansing.

Example - As I look out my window, I see soul-stirring scenes reminiscent of James Russell Lowell's descriptive *The First Snow Fall* — his "stiff rails softened to swan's down," — his trees with "ermine too dear for an earl," — and his poorest twig on the elm tree "inch deep with pearl."

Why soul stirring? Every year at the first big snowfall, I am reminded of Lowell, who captured in words a snow scene as picturesque as any painting. Then I remember his lines about his daughter, Mabel – who "could not know my kiss was given to her sister, folded close under deepening snow" – and I have a good healthy cry, tears streaming down my face. What a relief!

Tears have replaced "painful lumps in my throat" — the way I used to grieve. How and when did I stop crying by blocking tears and grief in my throat? How did I finally unblock the energy?

Bear with me as I describe a few pieces of my puzzle. For years I buried seemingly unrelated memories until physical trauma (an automobile accident, pesticide poisoning, natural gas leak and oil leak) turned a healthy athlete into an invalid with life-threatening Environmentally Triggered Illness (ETI).

Soul Searching revealed and eventually released my blocked energy, which helped me to heal. Until I made the connection, I didn't realize that I was living with a sinkhole that was draining positive energy from my well-being.

Good Intentions but Inappropriate Shielding Reared in a happy, closely knit family, I was taught to be sensitive to others' feelings. For instance, my father always cautioned us not to cry in front of my mother "because crying upsets her." Once when Dad was driving me home from school, he had a digestive attack with pain so severe he had to stop the car. He admitted to me that he had been experiencing these attacks for a few weeks, but "DON'T TELL MOMMA, IT WILL UPSET HER." I did as he asked.

Blocking My Tears Three weeks later, as I sat next to Mom going to my father's funeral, I had this terrible pain in my throat as I held back my tears and kept thinking, "Daddy, see I'm not crying."

A few years later, at the funeral of my two-year-old niece, Barbie, I again choked my tears in my throat, "to protect Momma." As an afterthought, what a shame! My crying might have helped Mom cry, unleashing her pent-up negative energy. Certainly crying would have allowed me to release a deeply held tension that caused me to have trouble with my throat whenever I was under heavy emotional or toxic stress.

♪♪♪♪♪

Retrospective More than learning to cry, Soul Searching can be learning to laugh again by allowing yourself to feel the depth of your emotions and feelings of your heart, positive as well as negative.

Notice that your abilities to feel pain and happiness are interdependent. People who are afraid to experience sadness and want to feel only happiness are fooling themselves. To appreciate a full measure of emotional response, you must be prepared to experience a full range of physical and emotional sensations — in other words, the movement of the Accordion.

Likewise, people who suffer the physical pain of chronic illness (including ETI) and protectively block that pain also inadvertently deprive themselves from experiencing love, happiness and Body Awareness.

♪♪♪♪♪

Dr. Kailin's Hypothesis From information my allergist, Dr. Kailin, gave me years ago, I now understand the impact of my funeral experience on my ETI. Using Hans Selye's[2] theory of stress (that the stress mechanism is equally activated by emotional/interpersonal stress as by physical stress), Dr. Kailin hypothesized that a stressful emotional response releases chemicals stored in body fat tissues, resulting in physical reactions. The body's reaction is virtually the same whether reacting to emotional or toxic stress. When combined with emotional or chemical/physical stressors, reactions become more acute.

Dr. Kailin's hypothesis also illustrates how blocked feelings created actual physical tension in the area associated with the failure to express my feelings. Often light pressure on these areas will lead to reliving the events and allow the tension to be released.

248

Since Dr. Kailin concluded that the main target of stress was the weakest organ at the time of the insult, why did I block in my throat? Why not my liver? Dad died of cancer of the liver, but more about that later.

CONTINUOUS PROCESSING

Processing occurs in bits and pieces. Now, return to my beautiful snow scene, an example of one step of a processing which can unblock long-forgotten traumas. Wilhelm Reich, a psychiatrist, labeled the negative accumulation of energy as "armoring of the body;" energy practitioners use the term "blocked energy." (See PROCEDURE below.)

As you will see below in "Natalie's Reign of Terror," I cited the snowfall to illustrate the value of Soul Searching and how it gave me closure. Now when nature occasionally duplicates Lowell's scene, my tears offer me closure that I missed over 40 years ago. I can peacefully feel spirits present and I can let Dad and Barbie "rest in peace."

As I reread this chapter in final preparation to send to the publisher, we are having a huge snowstorm.

I realize how different I am now whenever I experience a snowstorm. I am now able to condition myself with positive memories – memories of playing in the snow with my father, playing "fox and geese" and sledding down a hill.

I see beautiful little Barbie smiling, playing in the snow. I watch her pounding the piano keys and listen to her "music" – beautiful treasures of cacophony.

My tears of pain are becoming cries of joy, and my throat has started to open up.

Once memories come alive, they flow in a beautiful stream. I remember holding my father's hand as we walked to services on the Sabbath. I remember the pride in my father's eyes and how he always bragged about me — I could outrun the boys; play softball, volleyball and basketball as well as any boy; and defeat anyone in ping-pong. I can see the smile on Barbie's face as she responded to hugs and kisses.[i]

Although initially my Soul Searching was very painful, my crying turned a negative into a positive, giving me relief by unblocking my THROAT Chakra. However, for proper progression of the learning process, first read about a less traumatic soul cleansing.

SPONTANEOUS PROCESSING INDUCED BY AN ODOR

I am sensitive to mold. Even when my sense of smell was impaired, I used to smell one type of mold that made me uneasy. I never knew why. Then, one time I was half listening to an old "Mash" rerun. In the show, the odor of a very moldy laundry bag sent Hawkeye (Alan Alda) into a sneezing attack, and he started a Soul Search for causes.

As usual, television typically solved a serious trauma in a half-hour program, but I began to think of my mold problem. During my next meditation, without any conscious plan, my Mind/body/soul/spirit spontaneously carried me back to a minor childhood fear I experienced on Halloween night. The eerie sounds, the weird lighting and a frightening tale occurred in a home that I now recall had that same mold odor.[3]

♪♪♪♪

```
Talk about negative conditioning!
```
♪♪♪♪♪

---

[i] I discovered that my two related emotional scars left me so confused that my pleasant memories were also co-mingled. Notice I intentionally did not edit this paragraph of memories. The words you read are what I just felt.

♪♪♪♪♪

Unfortunately, when emotional distress occurs in polluted environments, many mild traumas do have serious repercussions. When traumas occur or phobias are created, the various associations that are connected with the scene will trigger the same fear, like the smell of mold taking me back to a scary scene on Halloween. Unfortunately, very often there is no conscious memory of the association without Soul Searching.

♪♪♪♪♪

Internalizing the Processing Each time you complete a processing to decondition a trauma and eventually internalize your soul cleansing, spend time practicing relaxation and meditation, Playing with your Aura© and grounding yourself.

♪♪♪♪♪

After I have taught the following procedure to patients, many of them later report success in speeding up their processing. Whenever they find it difficult to get rid of a pain after they have grounded themselves, they concentrate on the pain and make a mental note to recall a time in which that pain was first locked into the body. Some also find that light pressure on the site of pain will create a flashback to the cause.

♪♪♪♪♪

Often energy is unblocked and pain disappears without recognition of a past trauma. Other times, however, people gain an insight into a past experience affecting their lives. That is soul cleansing at its best. It is especially effective when you have experienced an insight into some environmental or physical trauma or a religious, spiritual or mental ordeal.

The internalizing process demonstrates the validity of the **Accordion Reserve**© model. Each time you internalize the process, you gain insight and release more locked tension in your body, thereby increasing your reserve. The need for unity of **Mind/body/soul/spirit** illustrates our title, *Energy – the Essence of Environmental Health.*

NATALIE'S REIGN OF TERROR

♫♫♫♫

Sunday, February 28, 1999, 4:30 a.m. I run to my kitchen and slam both doors shut.

Stream of Consciousness Why don't I feel safe? Was I meditating? Was it a dream? How creepy. Wind on my face, wind at my back, wind above my head! What was that whirling sound? Was that really a bat I saw in my bedroom?

Can't stop shivering, teeth chattering, insides trembling, and sweating, shivering, cold. Why can't I force myself to go upstairs to get a blanket? Am I going into insulin shock again? Is my hypoglycemia returning? No, no, had no sugar. Maybe I need protein anyway. I'll eat some nuts. Can't swallow nuts - gag - throat closed up. Can't scream, can't talk, have no voice. Can't call for help. Throat hurts, stomach pains.

CALM YOURSELF, NATALIE! MEDITATE!

7:30: Calmer now. Eating breakfast. Healing meditation helped. My voice is back. I can swallow my food — My thoughts seem rational. I'm okay, that wasn't a bat. It was a dream. OH! NO! There is a bat in my kitchen!

7:45: Upstairs in guest bedroom, door slammed shut. Called 911, called Humane Society. Waiting for help.

Stream of Consciousness Shivering, feel crawly all over. Can't control teeth chattering. Throat closes up again. No wonder they couldn't understand me. Are there two bats? How did they get through closed doors? Two bats? More? Where are they coming from?

RELAX, NATALIE, MEDITATE

Comment The rest of Sunday seems very vague. I remember the man from the Humane Society. I remember my relief when he found only one bat. I also remember, however, the fear I experienced when he recommended I have someone investigate to be sure I did not have a family of bats living in my attic. But why did I cover my head when I ran downstairs to open the door for the man when he left?

I spent the day meditating, relaxing, healing and soaking in a tub of hot water with 2 cups each of Epsom salts and baking soda,[i] followed by a cleansing shower. I was finally calm enough to fall asleep in the guest room, the one furthest from my bedroom.

When I awoke Monday morning, the terror was gone but I was still uneasy. I kept wondering why I had covered my head before returning to my own bedroom. Why did I push the door slightly ajar and reach in along the wall to turn on the light switch? It was daylight — I didn't need a light.

I wouldn't call it fear. It was the same uneasy tension I have always felt at a mystery movie, an occasional familiar tension that I could never fathom. I knew I had to take time off then and there to process the experience.

PROCEDURE OF PROCESSING EMOTIONAL/PHYSICAL TRAUMAS

<u>Soul Searching</u> — *Very Personal Experience* Meditation/Relaxation, Grounding, Body Awareness (connecting a pain with

---

[i] A "detox bath" – it's like a natural spa.

an emotion), Stream of Consciousness, Deconditioning and Reconditioning are the foundations of Soul Searching.

You've succeeded in each phase on your path to healing, but we won't "quiz you on it." What follows are the steps I used to help me through my fears and tension. Follow your body's instincts as I followed mine.

Meditation Seated comfortably in a rocking chair in my living room, my eyes closed to avoid visual distraction, I meditated for thirty minutes. (Refresh your memory by reviewing Chapters 7-12.)

Body Awareness As I began to think about the fear, my throat again began to hurt. Connecting my fear and pain, I repeated many times: "My Mind/body/soul/spirit is taking me back to times when I blocked fear in my throat." As I concentrated on my throat, my pain intensified.

As I regressed, my emotions and pain were as intense, if not more so than what I experienced Sunday. The tightness in my throat once again made me aware of how we hold past traumas in our bodies, in our muscles. The holding pattern in turn makes us chronically tense and thereby depletes our Accordion Reserve©. As I put these events in print, I strengthen the effect of my Soul Searching.

Stream of Consciousness — First Flashback Abbreviated and minus the deep emotional and physical pain I experienced, I'll provide you just enough content to illustrate to you how my Mind/body/soul/spirit led me into a stream of consciousness of different fears that were somehow connected.

Alone with six-year-old niece Cindy, baby-sitting, watching TV, there is a face in the window — mustn't scream — I'll frighten her — take her into kitchen for a snack. Terrified — horrible face in windows — hard to be calm. Can't eat — can't swallow. Is window locked? Can't return to room.

254

Meditation - Relaxation - Grounded The procedure takes longer than usual for Autonomatic Pilot to kick in because the fear is so intense.

Comment Please note between each flashback the emotion became so stressful that it was a strain on my immune system. Each time I stopped to meditate, relax and practice grounding. I did not go back into the fear again until I could release the stress. Each time Autonomatic Pilot kicked in more quickly until finally all I had to do was keep thinking "Autonomatic Pilot" as I took three relaxation breaths and Autonomatic Pilot kicked in, freeing me to continue.

Summary of Stream of Consciousness — Second Flashback Next day, my brother Abe and I were visiting cousin Marian. "Marian, there's a bat in the hallway." Abe laughs — "Nat sees things — yesterday a peeping Tom, today a bat — Oh, she did see a bat. Look Marian, a bat is flying back and forth from your kitchen to your guest bedroom!"

Meditation - Relaxation - Grounding Relieved my fear of remembered bat.

Third Flashback I'm nine years old — look on window sill to see clock — FACE in the window — run to my father sleeping on the couch — jump on couch to be near him — startle Daddy — instinctively throws out his arm —- catches me in throat —- throws me on the floor — Daddy cradles me in his arms — throat hurts — can't cry — Daddy hurt me.

Fourth Flashback I'm eight years old — older friend and I reading forbidden mystery pulp romance novel — feel guilty — terrified as I read of a bat becoming entangled in the bride's veil. Meditation relieved tension.

Deconditioning

As stated above, between each flashback, I meditated using breathing, grounding, visualization, Playing with My Aura© and Automatic Pilot to relax me and remove stress. Fortunately, we do not have to relive the experience over and over to decondition the trauma, but we can do so using our imagination, remembering and relaxing.

When I was ready, I began to decondition each previous flashback. As an example of my procedure for your guideline, I shall use the fourth flashback:

As soon as I was totally grounded and relaxed, totally at peace, I visualized myself watching a movie about the peeping Tom. This time, I wrote my own scenario, letting my imagination run wild so my memories would be pleasant.

Visualization See the peeping Tom, run to Daddy for comfort, jump on Daddy, bumping my throat on the arm of the couch. I begin to cry. "Daddy, I hurt myself." Daddy cradles me in his arms, comforts me. Tells me something cold will ease the pain. Gives me big dish of chocolate ice cream. (Yes, I'm a reformed chocoholic, but visualization is a good way to get my chocolate goodies without abusing my body.) Throat feels good. I have no trouble swallowing. Daddy takes me by the hand and leads me to the hall. See a Halloween "trick or treater" wearing a mask. Give him a treat. Daddy and I have a good laugh.

Reconditioning Whenever my throat hurts and I cannot swallow, I repeat three times: "My Mind/body/soul/spirit will remind me to breathe, relax and remember how soothing the cold ice cream felt and how peaceful and calm I was when Dad cradled me." I go on Automatic Pilot, feel grounded and spend a few minutes healing my THROAT Chakra. Not only does my throat relax, but I become less reactive to the toxins.

BENEFITS OF SOUL SEARCHING – THE BAT TRAUMA

Emotional The fear, although so blocked in my body, never before had manifested itself. Was the Soul Searching worth it? After my bat incident and my Soul Searching, I visited with my cousin Marian and reminded her of the bat. In fact, Marian told me she has since had two more incidents with bats in that bedroom. I slept there like a baby for the five nights of my visit.

Physical I reinforced my ability to release current and future grief traumas by crying instead of blocking my THROAT Chakra. I have even had success using my Automatic Pilot after my beloved cousin Marian died. Circumstances beyond my control kept me from attending her funeral, but I was able to share a good healthy cry when I wrote my "Celebration of Marian's Life" and talked to Marian's surviving sister.

Insights I now understand the frequent blocking of my THROAT Chakra. As an adult, going back into the incident, I can recall my dad's contrition when he struck out his arm, caught me in the throat and threw me to the floor. I can recall how he hugged me and tried to explain he was sleeping and startled when I "flew" into the room and jumped on him. My body, however, had formerly remembered only the pain in my throat, the fear and the shock of having my loving, caring father hurt me.

In a sense, I have revealed a very personal, private Soul Searching to help you with your insights. You too may be unaware of an intense trauma. I never realized how I kept blocking fear. I always found excuses for certain idiosyncrasies:

* Avoiding mystery stories by rationalizing that "tension is unhealthy for everyone"
* Missing Hitchcock's *The Birds* because even the commercial made me tense

     *   Always being uneasy at night near windows, checking and pulling curtains together very close "because I value my privacy"

None of these idiosyncrasies seriously affected my life-style. However, little things mean a lot; each tense moment caused a shrinking of my Accordion Reserve©.

PROCESSING WITH HELP

Sometimes, it is helpful to explore a disturbing flashback with someone who has had training in processing. Once I was demonstrating my latest grounding procedure to Alan. In his own words below, Alan will describe his experience and how it has affected him. Processing was the furthest thing from our thoughts. I was merely teaching Alan my system of grounding.

I started by leading Alan through the SHORTCUT (PHASE III) and Grounding (Chapter 11) and reminded him to use my words only if necessary to keep him focused on positive thoughts and visualizations. Although Alan was vaguely aware of my voice and words, as soon as he reached his Awakening his own visualization took over. He began showing signs of spontaneous processing.

At this point I want to emphasize that I was not acting as Alan's therapist; I was merely a catalyst. With his permission I responded to his words, actions and pains – nothing more.

When Alan's throat tightened and I could see he was having trouble swallowing, I suggested he concentrate on his throat and intensify his discomfort. When he began to complain in a whisper, I suggested he give voice to his words, speak louder as if he meant it. When he complained of pain in his leg and kept asking why he was being held down, it was then that I sat on his leg to restrain it.

♪♪♪♪♪

258

ALAN'S VERSION

♫♫♫♫♫

Comment Natalie asked me to write my recollec-
tions of my *Soul Searching* from my "novice days." I intentionally did not read Natalie's version, nor did I discuss it with her, before I wrote what follows. Since my
experience occurred so many years ago, I wanted to discover how much I really remembered.

So Much Pain I Could Feel It In my early practice
of *Meditation/Relaxation* with Natalie, I was aware that I
was not well-balanced. By using comparisons, I
discovered that my entire right leg would not vibrate
and tingle like my other leg and arms would.

My awareness extended to injuries I sustained to
my right leg (hip and thigh) during my marathon training
4-5 years before. I recalled that my right 3rd toe sustained a stress fracture about 2-3 years later.

As my image paths connected, I recalled that my
right hip always gave me difficulty when I tried to swim
– especially the frog kick. The memories came back, but
the energy flow through my right hip and leg remained
blocked.

I visualized running and swimming, and I began to
feel pain in my right hip. I felt my energy move up and
through my upper chakras, and I sensed that my larynx
was tight.

Natalie encouraged me to sing or speak. My throat
felt paralyzed and constricted. I remained silent. I felt
tense.

I returned to images of energy coursing through my
CROWN Chakra to my feet and hands and then back up
again. My right foot would tingle when energy flowed upward, but energy would not traverse my right hip, nor my
THROAT Chakra.

After what seemed like an eternity, I suddenly
found myself crying uncontrollably – sobbing, gasping –
tears flowing, nasal passages congested, neck and face
sweating. My right leg felt dead, and there was intense
pain in my right hip.

259

These sensations were both startling and terrorizing. I was frightened, but I was unable to voice my fear. I felt trapped. Natalie reminded me that I could retreat to safety any time I wanted by using the SHORT-CUT.

I returned to my energy image flowing from my CROWN Chakra to my feet and back up to my CROWN Chakra. I sensed the residual "dead" right leg and hip, but my larynx was less tense. I recall "wrapping myself" in a mummy-like cocoon for protection. A sense of calm returned.

I embarked on another round of discomfort and distress – much the same as the first. But this time I had a bit more confidence that I would recover. Nevertheless, I was soon overwhelmed by the same dread as before. In the midst of my turmoil, I still needed Natalie to guide me to safety.

I must have experienced another two or three lurches at some unseen and unrecognized trap that kept my right leg pinned to the mat. Each approach was full of sobbing, buckets of tears and lots of Kleenex. Every recovery came more easily.

Yet I was stymied – still no awareness of "why" I felt my right leg anchored to the mat. And, like all insights, the image suddenly appeared amidst tears, gulps for air and pain! I was at my circumcision – a mere eight days old. Family members were all around, holding my legs, as the moyel performed the ceremonial cuts.

Despite my agony, I felt incredible relief, as tears of pain turned to tears of joy. I was now able to move my leg. Energy flowed up and down – from my soles to my crown and beyond and down again.

I revisited my peaceful state and then exited with mixed thoughts. Did I really experience my own circumcision? I was very skeptical. I knew that Natalie had never suggested any images to "lead me." So I contacted my mother. Mothers always remember details of such important events. I told her who was standing around me, and she confirmed that I had correctly identified five of my six relatives.

What is the significance of my Soul Searching? For the first time, I was finally able to initiate a full recovery program for my right leg and hip. I had always performed appropriate exercises and stretches, but complete healing always eluded me. I can report that I have had no further injuries to my right leg.

"And Now You Know the Rest of the Story" Thanks again to Paul Harvey for this phrase. Notice how my experiences and flashbacks paralleled Natalie's, and that mine actually preceded hers chronologically. Notice also one small detail that I omitted from my memory – Natalie was pinning my leg down, but not until after I was already crying out that my leg was pinned down! Her action only assisted me to sense the image, which I had blocked for a lifetime.[i]

♪♪♪♪

Changing and Embellishing the Procedure Notice how Alan used my procedure, changing and embellishing my processing, using his Body Awareness, his visualization, his stream of consciousness. Later I borrowed from Alan what is comfortable for me.

You do the same, using as a guideline the abbreviated procedure I followed to unblock the childhood traumas, which erupted when the bat entered my room (see above).

WHERE AND WHEN TO SEEK HELP

We have found over the years that the body will release emotions only after you are comfortable with the process and are ready to proceed. If, as a novice, you run into deep emotions, seek professional help capable of playing the catalyst. My mentor, Dr. James Cox,[ii] followed the school of thought that to be capable of guiding patients through Soul Searching, one must first experience personal Soul Searching. Let that be a guide in choosing professional help.

♪♪♪♪

---

[i] The catalyst that Natalie supplied – holding down my leg – was not part of my own life experience. The catalyst did not initiate the imaging sequence, but instead intensified the power of the image. That is most likely why I didn't recall it as I wrote my version.

[ii] James Cox, Dr. theol.

Shielding Certain reactions or blocking emotions, which seemed right at the time based on one's understanding of the state of affairs, with later insight from Soul Searching, will frequently reveal well-intended but inappropriate shielding. We develop behavioral habits in certain ways because of repetition of actions we learned. Soul Searching can help you undo inappropriate actions and traumas resulting from well-meaning but apparently unintentional shielding.

♫♫♫♫♫

Sleep and Shielding Recall from Chapter 13: "Conditioning" my recommendations on helping infants sleep "8 hours at 8 weeks." Sometimes infants continue to wake up, and parents wonder why they are unsuccessful in promoting baby's continuous sleep. They sometimes ignore the "problem," and accept it as a mark of their sustained fatigue ("Fog Heads" in Chapter 13). I often explain the following situation to mom, who is most often involved, since she has to wake up to nurse, unless it is dad who occasionally offers the bottle.

Baby wakes crying to be fed. Mom quickly greets the wake-up cry by nursing, and the crying ceases. This action provides inadvertent positive reinforcement for crying and further encourages future wake-ups. I recommend allowing baby to cry until he really needs to be fed, at which time mom should offer to do the business of feeding but not give the attention.

Why does mom go to nurse baby so quickly when it would be more desirable to discourage attention at this time? The answer is "shielding" or protection.

Mom's perception is that somebody will wake up because baby is crying. So silencing baby's cry quickly "protects" someone from also waking – an older sibling, dad (who has to get up early to go to work), grandma (down the hall) or a neighbor (in an adjoining apartment).

Another "shielding" occurs if mom had to return to work after maternity leave. Feeling "guilty" about not spending time with baby, she now finds comfort in the nurturing she provides during this nighttime encounter. Unknowingly she is "protecting" herself.

In other childhood sleep disturbance situations, I have discovered that parents had experienced their own sleep disturbances as toddlers. Believing they were comforting the crying toddlers, the parents were actually protecting themselves because they had never done their own Soul Searching.

This sleep disturbance is a classic example of negative conditioning for baby, mother and family. The intentions are well meaning but have an adverse impact on everyone. You can clearly see how some sleep disturbances become generational.

♫♫♫♫♫

From clinical experiences, we have found that you cannot compartmentalize emotional responses; they involve Mind/body/soul/spirit. When you are well grounded and your Accordion Reserve© is high, you react to a lesser degree than when your reserve is depleted. That's just one plus! Even more important is the natural processing that occurs during Meditation/Relaxation and grounding in a similar way that dreams automatically process traumas.

Once you have recognized Your Awakening which is the awareness of your body's sensations in its most relaxed and grounded state you will learn to recognize little signs and symbols which are gateways to your soul. In reality, you have such signs all the time. The meditative state merely amplifies your awareness.

SUMMARY - PATHS TO SOUL SEARCHING

"The Road Not Taken" [4] As a protective mechanism to help you function during a crisis, you stow physical or emotional "baggage" as suppressed negative (blocked) energy. Until processed, your negative energy can resurface over your life's journey as recurrent physical or emotional symptoms, triggered by, for example, pesticide exposure, an automobile accident, a running injury or the death of a child.

Many health care professionals debate whether illness is physically or psychologically (emotionally) induced. We find that there need not be a controversy. As we worked with the autonomic nervous system and the model of the Accordion Reserve©, we were able to conclude that illness is a composite of physical and psychological factors. They are inseparable in any discussion of promoting healing and Environmental Health.

From examples described in this chapter, you can observe that:

* Physical (body-based) signs and symptoms of disease are frequently triggered by biological/chemical/physical factors.
* Body-based signs and symptoms of illness may also be triggered by emotional factors.
* Emotional (mind-based) signs and symptoms may be triggered by mind/soul/spirit factors.
* Mind-based signs and symptoms may be triggered by biological/chemical/physical factors.

"The Road Not Taken" Some day conscious Soul Searching will become the preferred path to help promote Environmental Health.

---

[1] John 8:32, New Testament, King James Version.
[2] Selye H. 1976. Forty years of stress research: principal remaining problems and misconceptions. *Canadian Med Assoc J*l 115:53-56.
[3] Smith CJ, Scott SM, Ryan BA. 1999. Cardiovascular effects of odors. *Toxicol Ind Hlth* 15: 593-601.
[4] Frost R. "The Road Not Taken."

21
ENHANCING YOUR SPIRITUAL BEING –
Spiritual Awareness Unifies Mind/body/soul/spirit

Prologue

Spiritual Dimension in Health There are two ways of defining Spiritual Healing. One is to use spiritual energies for healing. Examples would be prayers and laying on of hands. The other way is to heal the disconnect between self and spiritual nature. In what follows, we focus on the role of using one's spiritual beliefs and practices in healing and the deepening or awakening of the spiritual dimension, which can become another force in eventual healing of self and others.

Ubiquitous Spirituality Throughout the ages, civilizations have used various terms to define their spiritual belief system. To name just a few: Supreme Force, Universal Unknown, the Native Americans' Creator Spirit, Buddha, Guiding Force, Allah and the Christian/Judaic term God. Whatever makes you comfortable, adopt the term from your belief; we shall be using the term God for our belief system. Whenever we use the term "God," substitute the term for your belief system.

Some of us believe the Creator is everywhere and in everything, including us humans. Although we find a higher sense of our spiritual being in houses of worship, both of us feel a bond with God and our energy in everyday individual pursuits and especially when we are working with patients. This spiritual awareness increases during our brainstorming sessions when we share our individual experiences. For us, the spiritual aspect of a person is the ubiquitous presence of God.

From the Old Testament: "And let them make ME a sanctuary that I may dwell among them."[1] From the New Testament come two verses: "Don't you know that you yourselves are God's temple and that God's spirit lives in you?"[2] and "Perfect love casteth out fear."[3]

When there is no fear, we are aware of our unity with God. Therefore the path to God is very closely related to the path to health, since fear depresses the immune system and intensifies allergies and makes us more vulnerable to disease. To be healthy is to be whole, and in almost all traditions, God is defined as One. True healing is therefore to be one with God. When we are one with God, the power of spiritual healing can be directed to heal others and ourselves.

Whatever your belief system is, whether it is oriented to house of worship, specific religion, humanism, spirit, culture, tradition, lifestyle or none of the above, we will show how working with your spiritual nature will increase your **Accordion Reserve**©.

Even in this very private relationship with our Creator, we are opening our souls, revealing very personal experiences in our attempt to teach by example. As with every other aspect of healing, use our spiritual examples and those of patients merely as guideposts to lead you into your own spiritual experiences. You may wish to carry what you learn into your house of worship, spiritual meeting place or under the trees and stars.

♪♪♪♪

In my search for a cure, I investigated any and every system that could add to my recovery. I knew my faith was so strong that nothing could lead me astray. On the contrary, my quest strengthened my faith in my own religious teachings. Patients report to me that they can adapt my procedures to strengthen their own beliefs, although theirs may differ from mine.

♪♪♪♪♪

ENHANCING YOUR SPIRITUAL BEING

There is controversy especially within the ranks of "by the book" mainstream medicine about the role of faith in medicine. In this section, we are in agreement with those who see an important role for faith in the process of healing. The usual questions we hear are:

*Are churchgoers healthier than non-churchgoers?

> Since some churchgoers are not necessarily spiritual, there is no way to research the questions, but we have seen for ourselves how patients have made more rapid progress when they have had a viable faith to assist them in facing their health problems. Limited research in this area supports our conclusion.[4]

*Is there any truth to miracle healing stories passed down through the ages?

> The answer is always "yes" if you ask a person who feels that the spiritual energies played a role in getting well and "no" if the starting point of the researcher is agnostic or the researcher demands scientific blind study research.

*What effect, if any, does the spiritual state of a patient have on healing processes?

> It is well established that faith in a doctor or in a medicine greatly enhances the effectiveness of treatment. If placebos owe their power to faith, then how much more power is there when the belief is grounded in devotion and faith in a divine source of healing?

We have always felt a spiritual effect on our energy and observed the same in our patients. However, we began a serious study of the energy/faith connection after a personal shared experience.

♪♪♪♪

High Holy Days Air quality in the sanctuary was more toxic than usual: windows closed, residue of mothball odors on clothes, perfume and aftershave overpowering. I began having trouble breathing, developing stinging eyes and distorted vision.

I closed my eyes and had difficulty doing breathing exercises, so I sat quietly, meditating, visualizing my aura and a garden with fresh, clean breezes. After a brief time, my head began to clear, my energy perked up and I felt grounded. I thought it was merely the effect of my meditation. However, when I opened my eyes to test my vision, I could see Alan focusing on his aura, directing his hands toward me and continuing without any break in his chanting. I began focusing on my aura to augment the spiritual energy he was sending me.

I was able to continue with the service despite the toxic atmosphere. During a brief break in the service, Alan's wife, Ruth, whispered to us, "You concentrate on your energies even in Temple?"

Especially in Services !!! Thanks to Ruth, we added a new dimension to healing. Our energy was not a distraction to our prayers, but an enhancement. In addition, if Ruth sensed our strengthened energy, what about congregants near us?

Observations Between prayers Alan and I unobtrusively focused on our auras and observed and sensed a surge of energy in the auric field of our neighbors as we grounded ourselves.

* Greatest increase was in the auric field of people nearest to us. During the holiest prayers, the auric fields increased in others even at a distance.
* The Rabbi's aura increased during his sermons, and the Cantor's aura increased as he led the chanting with the congregation.

* The more we focused on sensing our auric fields and projecting them towards others, the stronger we felt, and the prayers had a more meaningful effect on us.

I used to say: "I no longer hear music, I feel it." Since I have experienced the Accordion Reserve©, *I realize that what I feel are musical vibrations.* Any sensory input generates a spiritual energy in my aura – when I see colorful art, taste and smell pure food and breathe pristine air.

♪♪♪♪

Once you become aware of the power of your energy, you are continually increasing your contact and connection with nature and other people. You are likely to sense the meaning of the greeting among Buddhists: "I greet the Buddha within you."

PERSONAL SPIRITUAL EXPERIENCE

♪♪♪♪

Vague Memories of Details - Stream of Consciousness (My apologies to my Native American friends if I have distorted the facts.) Sweat lodge on a farm four hours away from home. Ceremony conducted by Native American — see someone building a huge bonfire — everyone filing into a huge enclosed tent through a flap door and sitting in a circle around a huge pile of heated stones — occasionally adding hot burning stones carried in on the burning hot tines of a pitchfork — taking turns throwing what looks like herbs before adding more heated stones — someone pouring water over the burning hot stones, sizzling hot steam engulfs us — my ears clogging, cannot hear words, but beginning to respond to chanting.

Vivid Memory - Stream of Consciousness My turn to throw herbs — hand pressed against burning hot pitchfork — smell burning flesh — that's my flesh burning — feel faint — intense pain — someone offers to take me out — thanks, but no — no — I'll be all right — don't disrupt the ceremony —

hand is hot — air so hot — gasping, can't breathe — sweat pouring down my face — my whole body — must meditate — must freeze my hand — visualize hand in ice — begin to shiver — in a daze — chanting voices like prayer — strange feeling — the tent feels filled with light — I'm not with group but I'm feeling their closeness — rather soothing — feel I must turn to God — feel God's presence — oh, thank you, God — no pain — can't feel the heat — can't feel the steam — someone nudges me to let me know everyone is leaving.

Comment As I left the tent, running through the rain to the car, I looked at my hand — no sign of any burn — no blister — nothing — no pain. My first thought was self-congratulatory, excited that my procedure worked so well. Then I chastised myself for indulging a false ego. I was quiet on the way back to the house. I began to pray and thank God for His gift of healing.

Flashback As I reviewed the experience and what it meant, I felt myself returning to a retreat center where we were listening to Mozart's Requiem Mass. I was in a very relaxed state when suddenly the face of a ferocious wolf appeared. I was totally frightened and tried to convince myself I was dreaming, but the image became even more frightening when I suddenly realized that the wolf represented my fear of death.

Death The Requiem Mass included the "Sanctus" (translated "Holy") which reminded me of "Kadosh" in my tradition: "Holy. Holy. Holy." Suddenly I thought of the 23rd Psalm (23:4): "Yea, though I walk through the valley of the shadow of death, I will fear no evil, for Thou art with me." At that moment the wolf lost its power to frighten me. I knew that no matter what was to happen, God was with me. His presence would be with me in life and in death. The fear of death left me, and I felt the presence of God with a new intensity.

I felt an instant release of tension as I experienced this insight. I realized that my fear of death was triggering many of my symptoms. In fact, when I was near death in the hospital many years ago, I stored my fear to protect myself. In my meditative state this powerful wolf image gave me the strength to unblock the negative energy of that fear.

Becoming Whole The Requiem Mass flashback furnished a context for my experience in the sweat lodge. As I gasped for air, the threat of death seemed imminent. My Requiem meditation helped restore calm and feel God's presence and protection, even as I again faced "my wolf" – my shadow of death.

As a result of my experience I now accept that Spiritual Healing is the sense of overcoming separation from the spiritual. I believe we must at some point confront and overcome the fear that death can separate us from our spiritual self. Prior to that, almost any symptom takes on the added freight of belief that we will die from the exposure, even when this is not conscious.

Sensitivity and Fine-Tuning One of my teachers used to say that ETI patients are harbingers of the future. More sensitive to outside triggers, in general, we react with more symptoms. Perhaps this same sensitivity is what permits us to be more aware that God is with us and in us at all times and all places. For me, this awareness has sparked my interest in various spiritual healing traditions and their importance.

♪♪♪♪♪

No matter what you call your belief system, you merely have to tune into your own insights. Our most productive insights occurred during our joint meditative sessions, when we were playing with our auras, and we were at the height of our spiritual inspiration.

♪♪♪♪♪

Fundamentally - It's Faith Through many similar experiences as a teacher, I found that patients' faith and mine are interdependent in promoting health and healing. The more a patient becomes grounded and aware of a grounding force, the more rapidly progress occurs.

When patients know and appreciate that I have faith in God (my belief system) and that my current state of health is implicit in that faith, I find that patients feel more comfortable adding their own belief system into their healing and health-promoting experiences. While I have no statistical information, I have the sense that their progress accelerates when they can add this faith dimension to their grounding.[i]

♫♫♫♫

Faith Healing Feeling energy, receiving energy, organizing energy, balancing energy and grounding energy are lessons you have learned in this book. From this perspective, it is a logical extension that the ancient tradition of Laying on of Hands[ii] could be a means of healing. Whether such healing occurs instantaneously, miraculously or over time does not matter. The fact that you believe is fundamental.

SPIRITUAL EXPERIENCE REVISITED

♫♫♫♫

Having recently read *Coyote Medicine*[5] by Lewis Mehl-Madrona, M.D., I realize the full power of the sweat lodge when performed by a Native American medicine man. While my experience was not like the casual New Age experience Dr. Mehl-Madrona mentioned, it also did not reach the spiritual height as conducted by an experienced practitioner described in *Coyote Medicine*.

---

[i] The Accordion Reserve© would predict that it is difficult but not impossible to design any study that determines how fast or how few sessions an individual needs to improve. Factors like how much "stored baggage" (negative energy) at the time of presentation may be the influential first variable.

[ii] Mackereth P, Wright J. 1997. Therapeutic touch: nursing activity or form of spiritual healing? *Complementary Therapies in Nursing & Midwifery*. 3(4): 106-10. This article references Dolores Krieger's first book on *The Therapeutic Touch* (1979).

In retrospect, I understand that my healing, my closeness with God and my ethereal experience were enhanced when combined with the powerful healing of Native American methods. The experience strengthens our belief (Alan's and mine) that Native American Medicine, Eastern Medicine and Environmental Medicine can blend together with mainstream Western Medicine, thereby demonstrating the power of Mind/body/soul/spirit — and the Accordion Reserve© can be the guide.

As I read the chapter "Sacred Fire" in *Coyote Medicine* it was dejà vu – how Alan and I have been working our separate ways for 20 years, yet following a path as if we were collaborating spiritually. So it is with Dr. Mehl-Madrona. Alan and I would like to meet Dr. Mehl-Madrona to share our mutual experiences. Even as we come from such diverse backgrounds, we travel shared paths.

SIMILAR DESTINATIONS ALONG UNCOMMON PATHS

<u>*Dejà vu*</u> As I read *Eagle's Quest*[6] I again experienced the sensation that I was crossing paths, this time with author Dr. Fred Wolf. He searched for scientific truth through the physics of healing, as performed by the Native American medicine man. My search was for a cure for my ETI. I realized how often we traveled the same path.

PRACTICAL APPLICATIONS

<u>*The Power of a Child's Faith*</u> Because I am an experienced school teacher trained in stress reduction and environmental health, it is not unusual that the types of patients pediatricians refer are children afflicted with hyperactivity, learning disabilities, autism and other childhood illnesses that fall under the umbrella of ETI.

Dr. Vinitsky (Alan, my co-author) referred Mia as a patient because, in addition to other manifestations of ETI, Mia appeared to have an advanced case of Tourette's Syndrome, motor tics and loud oral tics. Mia's case deserves special attention because it fits so completely in this chapter. Mia's religious faith made it easier for her to accept the healing power that comes from God. It is a tribute to her parenting that Mia was so receptive.

First Impressions My first impression of Mia was of a very well-behaved, pretty eight-year-old child who sat still drawing detailed pictures. Notice I did not say quietly because Mia's oral tics were loud and squeaky and were accompanied by blinking of her eyes. Clearly she was a talented child.

Because this is being written only to illustrate the applications of the process, I will not discuss the Ecologic-Oriented History questionnaire, her medical history, or the questioning of Mia's mother that led me into the procedure with which I worked with Mia.

"Don't you know that God's spirit is within you?"[7]

As we were getting acquainted (becoming friends), we discussed the slogan on Mia's tee-shirt: "In God We Trust." We spoke of God's love and recited together from Corinthians: "Don't you know that you yourselves are God's temple and that God's spirit lives within you." That is what established a good relationship between the two of us.

Games, Not Lessons Using Simple Simon, a game that Mia liked, whenever I said the words "Simple Simon says 'do this,'" Mia and her mother followed the lessons of relaxation breathing as I went through the motions (see Chapter 7). I did not refer to any of the terminology such as "visualization" or "aura."

Once Mia was able to follow the instructions for breathing, I taught her to have fun by:

* Lightly tapping up and down her arms, legs and body
* Dancing, swaying her arms back and forth
* Pulling and pushing her arms
* Pretending that she was dancing with her feet and leading an orchestra with her hands

She had so much fun as she led the orchestra, I led her into a song that she knew, "Do a Deer.."[i] a song with six of the Chakra sounds. (See Chapters 10, 11 and 12.)

It was a joy to watch the enthusiasm and excitement of this pretty eight-year-old playing with her aura and describing that she felt her hands were pulling each other.[ii] I also showed her the eye exercises to "help her blinking eyes." These were the same as described in "Seeing Is Believing."

Since Mia has been raised and educated in a Christian day school, I told her: "Picture your feeling as the energy of God's light. God sends his energy to the magnetic fields around the earth and to all human beings.

* Just look at the light and think of your feeling.
* Use it and imagine.
* Put your hands up as if you are praying to God.
* Pull down the beautiful white light and the shield of God down through your eyes, then your throat, then your heart, until it reaches way down to the ground."

---

[i] Rogers R, Hammerstein O. "Do-Re-Mi" from "The Sound of Music."

[ii] At first, Mia didn't know what to call the feeling. Just as Alan described in "Terrible Two's" conditioning (Chapter 9), I asked Mia if she knew what magnets are. She then described a pair of magnets that were stored on the refrigerator. Then she connected the magnet sensation with the feeling between her hands. In other words, it is difficult for children to verbalize non-visual feelings, until someone can mirror the sensation.

"Let's play another game of Simple Simon," I suggested. I followed the pattern of the game with her, but for the sake of brevity, I omit each reference to Simple Simon.

* Pick up the energy that God put into the beautiful soil.
* Take the energy into your hands.
* Lift your hands, as if you are praying, and receive more of God's energy.
* Hold the energy in your hands.
* Slowly move your hands down the sides of your body.
* Put the energy into your hip pockets.

As with all my patients, I told Mia I take no credit for what she has accomplished, that it is a gift that God has given her. The gift was a true gift, a visible and an oral gift, because after just one lesson, she returned to see me two more times, and there were no other signs of a tic except some blinking that remained.

Because of the distance they have to travel and because her parents work and Mia has school, I have not seen her since the third lesson. However, her mother reports that as long as Mia avoids milk products (her worst allergy), and she practices her breathing and visualizations, the tics remain under control. Mia's mother said she would bring her back for more lessons once Mia gained more strength and could tolerate the long drives in heavy traffic.

Mia's success depended on faith, playing games and laughter. Whenever she performed better than her Mom, Mia and I formed an alliance, laughing and clapping with each "victory." In other words, her laughter, joy and zest for life facilitated her faith in Spiritual Healing.

♪♪♪♪

SUMMARY

Spiritual Healing is a:

* Sense of overcoming our separation from the spiritual.
* Flashback to infancy and childhood — when learning is a joyful game of practice and repetition.
* Rejuvenation, nourishment and fulfillment of the soul:
    * As you trust your Guiding Force to orchestrate Your Awakening.
    * Through patience and security.
    * With laughter, music, light and tears.
    * Without envy, conflict, anger or competition with yourself and others.

Spiritual Healing is a unification of Mind/body/soul/spirit.

---

[1] Exodus 25:8.
[2] Corinthians 3:16-17.
[3] I John 4:18 (King James).
[4] Matthews D. 1998. *The Faith Factor.* Penguin Books, New York.
[5] Mehl-Madrona L. 1997. *Coyote Medicine Lessons from Native American Healing.* Fireside, New York.
[6] Wolf FA. *Eagle's Quest.* 1992. Simon and Schuster Trade Paperbacks, New York.
[7] Corinthians 3:16-17.

EPILOGUE

Serendipity? Coincidence? Synchronicity? Is there a plan? Do we respond to a plan? Are we part of a plan? Do we create our own plan? Do we have choice? Or is it all pre-destined?

Such ethical questions have been the basis of philosophers' debates through the ages. We leave it to you to ask, to challenge, to grow and to heal. Forever, use the **Accordion Reserve**©. We hope you will be inspired.

PART VIII

The Model

PROFESSIONAL CHALLENGES

PROFESSIONAL
CHALLENGES
Posing Questions, Building on Learning, Changing Directions

Early Recognition of Autonomic Neuropathy

Prologue

Since you have turned to this chapter, you are interested in knowing some of the details of the Accordion Reserve© model and hypothesis. Chapter 5 introduces you to the model, while Chapter 6 highlights the link between the autonomic nervous system (ANS) and the Accordion. Chapters 7-12 teaches you Conditioned Breathing, Body Awareness and the power of energy, setting the stage for the next 9 chapters, which are devoted to developing Energy interrelationships.

Notice that we begin with sleep, followed by exercise and nutrition in Chapters 13-15. The interdependence of these energy generators is crucial to understanding the improvement of energy, healing and improving Environmental Health. In the current chapter we emphasize the power of relationships among these through complex communication processes.

In Chapters 16-18, we address environmental controls, improving our external environment — air, food and water in order to effect a change on our internal environment.

Finally, in Chapters 19-21, we teach using **Body Awareness** as a technique to discover the adverse effects on our internal energy. In Chapter 19 "Self-Testing," **Body Awareness** helps a person to discover what external factors (such as foods, air, water) may be contributing to symptoms. In Chapter 20 we offer our personal examples of discovering the impact of negative energy on recurring symptoms. As you will see, **Cleansing Your Soul** of that negative energy is a powerful means of expanding your Accordion. Finally, Chapter 21 emphasizes the benefits of having and using your **Belief System** to develop **Spiritual Healing** — creating unity of **Mind/body/soul/spirit**.

We welcome you in joining our discovery.

FOUNDATIONS OF MEDICINE REVISITED

♫♫♫♫♫

As a young medical student I learned that the foundation for superb diagnosis and treatment always begins with a history and physical. In today's environment of managed care, reimbursements discourage the essential component of quality health care — TIME!

It would be ideal if the patient would provide accurate and complete details without prompting from the listener. Yet the reality is that unless the questioner is prepared to seek new information in a unique format, the correct diagnosis will often be missed.

I am reminded of a recent patient who appeared quite intelligent, presented as somewhat hyperactive, and gave a history that lacked chronological organization. Despite having a long history of fibromyalgia and sensitivity to odors, she apparently lacked the insight to recognize that many of the recent changes in her workplace and living quarters were making her sick. She was hard working and dedicated to maintain her work so that she could keep her insurance. Yet she was trapped by her circumstances — doctors who didn't have the answers, employers who let her go and her limited financial resources to obtain a cure. Her lack of insight may have been driven out of necessity - denial so that she could make do.

In the Foreword of this book, I cited Dr. Gerdes' eulogy of Dr. Randolph. I return to Dr. Randolph's book *Human Ecology and Susceptibility to the Chemical Environment*.[1] Dr. Randolph stated that he was writing his book to describe the "chemical environment" and "secondarily with the resulting *clinical manifestations*" [his emphasis]. Yet it is his extraordinary description of manifestations, based on his power of observation, which sets the bar for us to emulate. I quote from page 21:

"As susceptibility to frequently encountered chemical exposures builds up, the process tends to spread to *related* materials to which exposures also exist. Adaptation to the total load gradually decreases, coincident with the onset of chronic symptoms.

"Chronic illness resulting from maladaptation to various parts of the chemical environment may manifest only as eye irritation, rhinitis, burning of the lips and skin, pruritus, bronchitis, mild gastrointestinal or other relatively minor symptoms, localized principally to major points of contact. For instance, if smog is the major exposure, eye irritation, running nose and coughing may be the principal symptoms, but if spray residues in foods are primarily involved, manifestations may be largely referable to the gastrointestinal tract.

"Later, more severe chronic respiratory symptoms may occur, including nasal obstruction, sinus involvement, severe coughing, and bronchial asthma; various dermatoses; a wide range of more troublesome gastrointestinal manifestations, and sometimes urgency and frequency of urination. Mild constitutional symptoms, such as physical and mental fatigue usually accompany the above chronic localized effects. These most frequently manifest as tiredness; a cut-back in former energy; lack of initiative and zest for work; forgetfulness; difficulty in thinking, concentrating and reading comprehension, and sometimes a relative impairment in the sense of humor. Other symptoms which often occur are headaches; various musculoskeletal aching and painful syndromes, including myalgia, fibrositis, bursitis, arthralgia and arthritis; neuritis and certain other neurological manifestations; and such other general effects as edema, palpitation, excessive perspiration, pallor and weakness.

"Localized manifestations tend to taper off in the presence of more advanced chronic constitutional syndromes. For instance, there is the chronic level of the so-called 'neuroses' characterized by more advanced mental confusion and mild depression. Although manifestations vary considerably, these include a tendency for fixed ideas, one-track thoughts and asocial attitudes; morose, sullen, seclusive, and sometimes hostile and paranoid behavior; negativeness to suggestion; and 'dopiness,' grogginess and an indifference to one's surroundings, sometimes approaching lethargy."

Dr. Randolph was describing symptoms of progressive autonomic neuropathy! I leave it to you to take the time, learn about the early manifestations of autonomic neuropathy and use the Accordion Reserve© model to reverse conditions before they become irreversible.
♫♫♫♫♫

PRINCIPLES OF OUR WORKING MODEL

The Accordion Reserve© model functions on two levels – 1) a descriptive, static mode and 2) a functional, dynamic mode.

The Descriptive Accordion - Static Mode reflects the current amount of energy in the organism; in other words the size of the Accordion. The influences on the size of the Accordion are its handles. The value of the static mode is to aid in diagnosis and treatment of conditions that result in dynamic Accordion dysfunction.

The Functional Accordion - Dynamic Mode operates on two planes – Energy and ANS.

* The Energy plane reflects the amount of energy added to or subtracted from the current state. As a stimulus, energy causes a respective increase or decrease in the size of the Accordion. This plane would be considered the stress.

* The ANS plane reflects the overall response (if any) of the body to the stimulus, which introduced the energy change. This description does not attempt to define specific reflexes or responses.

THE WORKING MODEL

Utility of a Working Model A working model should help diagnose illness, identify causes, recognize symptoms, direct treatment and improve health. Readers of all backgrounds are encouraged to explore the powerful implications of the **Accordion Reserve©**.

Descriptive Accordion As described by Dr. Randolph and reiterated by many observers subsequently, there is strong clinical evidence and anecdotal proof linking chronic low-dose or recurrent intermittent exposures of toxins to many conditions.[2] Logic and common sense fill gaps when scientifically reproducible evidence is hard to come by. Compare **Tables PC-1 and PC-2.**

ENVIRONMENTAL FACTORS	
EXTERNAL ENVIRONMENT	**INTERNAL ENVIRONMENT**
BIOLOGICAL	**ORGAN SYSTEMS**
Bacteria, Viruses, Molds, Parasites, Animals, Plants and their derivatives, etc.	Nervous, Cardiovascular, Gastrointestinal, Musculoskeletal, etc.
CHEMICAL	**ORGANS**
Inorganic, Organic, Metals, Solvents, Pesticides, Air Pollutants, Vapors, etc.	Liver, Heart, Lungs, Brain, etc.
	CELLS
	Skin, Muscle, Nerve, etc.
PHYSICAL	**CELL SUBSTRUCTURES**
Light, Sound, Barometric Pressure, Wind, Radiation, Gravity, Magnetic Fields, etc.	Nucleus, Mitochondria, Cell Membrane, DNA, RNA, Molecules, etc.

Table PC-1. Environmental Factors of the Descriptive Accordion. External and Internal Environmental Factors.

The Handles of the Accordion represent the descriptive triggers that might result in Environmentally Triggered Illness (ETI). The description would further represent potential therapies to reverse the triggers. Of course, therapies would be directed at any clinically identified specific triggers or mechanisms that are identified in the diagnostic phase.

Table PC-1 outlines environmental influences of the descriptive Accordion. These are both outside and inside the body. **Table PC-2** highlights energy factors. Notice that environmental factors in **Table PC-1** have a relationship with each other and are listed again in **Table PC-2** for that reason.

ENERGY FACTORS	
SLEEP	Quantity, Quality: Onset, Completion, Interruptions, Phase Shifts, Conditioning
EXERCISE	Quantity, Quality: Type, Timing, Intensity, Pattern, Conditioning
NUTRITION	Quantity, Quality: Selections, Contaminants, Supplements
RELATIONSHIPS	
Self	Self-image, Attitudes, Motivation, Moods, Sleep, Exercise, Nutrition
Others	Family, Friends, Peers, Superiors, the Public
External Environment	
Mode of Entry	Inhalation, Ingestion, Absorption through Skin, Sensory Input
Mode of Exit	Exhalation, Defecation, Urination, Sweating, Tearing, Secreting, Lactating, Bleeding, Physical Responses – crying, hitting
Internal Environment	Genetic, Enzymatic, Anabolic, Catabolic, Neural, Hormonal, Immunological
Guiding Force	Religion, Universal Energy
BELIEF SYSTEM	

Table PC-2. Energy Factors of the Descriptive Accordion.

In the descriptive, static mode the Accordion Bellows represents the accumulated effect of the triggers at any moment in time; in other words, the current state of an individual's energy. As illustrated in Chapter 5, an expanded Accordion represents Environmental Health, while a collapsed Accordion represents severe ETI. Of course, there is a broad spectrum between those two extremes.

Relationships of the External and Internal Environment Movement of the Handles of the Accordion depends on a series of communications. This is a transfer of information via energy management. **Figure PC-1** simplifies a communication sequence that could represent a "feedback loop." **Table PC-3,** which follows, highlights corresponding factors that facilitate communication relationships. An alteration may occur anywhere in the loop, but for simplicity, the components are listed 1 through 4. For example, a viral invader imitates a messenger that passes through a blood vessel, then arrives at a receptor that stimulates a nerve cell, which generates a neurotransmitter. In other words, one sequence influences a second, by any of the environmental factors listed in **Table PC-1.**

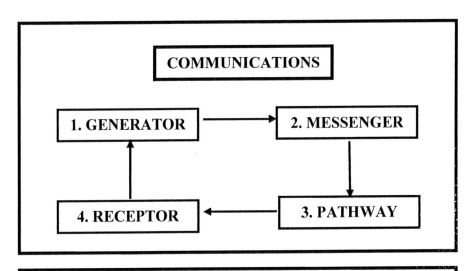

Figure PC-1. Communications in the Body. A stimulus creates a response in your body through a sequence of communications. The effect may be subtle or easily observable. An alteration may be introduced anywhere in the loop, resulting in a communication sequence.

| COMMUNICATIONS ||
1. GENERATOR	2. MESSENGER
Nerve Cells	Hormones
Glands	Neurotransmitters
Lymphocytes	Vibrations
Mitochondria	Molecules
Invaders	Imitators
4. RECEPTOR	**3. PATHWAY**
Messenger Specific	Blood Vessels
Non-specific	Nerves
Sensory Organs	Extravascular Space
	Meridians
	Membranes

Table PC-3. Communications Components – Some examples of Component Types.

Functional Accordion In addition to its descriptive static representation of an individual's energy, the Accordion Bellows changes size as it is continuously influenced by the complex interaction of its Handles. There are two planes — Energy and ANS.

Energy Input as an absolute value is added to the system. If added as an expenditure ("negative energy"), the Accordion Bellows shrinks. If energy is acquired, the result is "positive," and the Bellows expands. Energy input of any type is a stimulus and is regarded as a stress. This model is consistent with Selye's description of eustress (positive stress) and distress (negative stress). Sources of energy are derived from the Handles of the Accordion.

The ANS When needed, the ANS responds to energy inputs to the system. If energy expenditure occurs, an attempt at correction will be enacted by the parasympathetic nervous system (PSNS). Reciprocally, excessive input of energy will trigger the sympathetic nervous system (SNS) to respond.

The simplest illustration of this concept is found in **Figure PC-2**. Communications are necessary to effect a response from the stimulus.

The ANS is not always needed for a response, if the response mechanism is adequate to handle the stress. For example, if a fat-soluble pollutant is inhaled and is transported directly to the liver, it may be quickly metabolized to a water-soluble product for excretion. Or it might be exhaled directly.

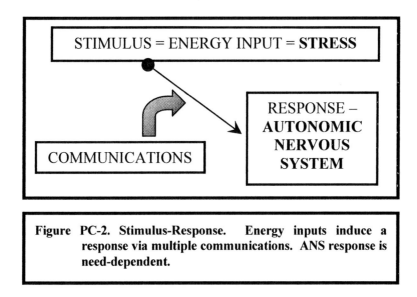

Figure PC-2. Stimulus-Response. Energy inputs induce a response via multiple communications. ANS response is need-dependent.

THE STRESS SPIRAL

♫♫♫♫♫

Early in my practice of medicine I composed a diagram that I now describe as the "Stress Spiral." At the time I was focusing on how to promote weight loss. However, the stress influence on the individual is plainly seen whether the complex response is cognitive, chemical or physiological. The Stress Spiral is illustrated in **Figure PC-3**.

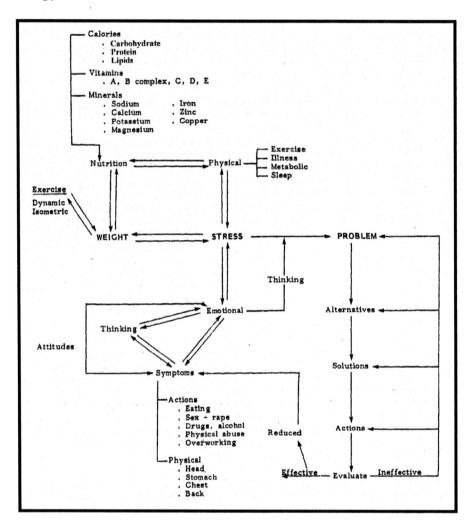

Figure PC-3. The Stress Spiral. Identifies the complex influences of stress on the individual.

Relationship with Self Explore the Stress Spiral for a moment. In it I tried to help patients understand what interfered with their ability to lose weight. Notice my former misguided emphasis on the cognitive aspects, which is still the tendency in medicine. "You could do it if you really wanted to," or so the saying goes.
♫♫♫♫♫

We now know that different physiologic disturbances, genetic predisposition and more, influence not only the success of a person's weight loss, but the consequences of that weight loss as well.

For example, a person sets a goal to lose weight for many reasons such as prevention or treatment of heart disease, diabetes, joint pain and arthritis, sleep apnea or chronic lung disease. But what happens if, after losing weight, a person develops chronic fatigue, chronic pain and mood changes?

It is proper attention to relationship with self that helps prevent these adverse consequences. As with any relationship, communications and energy factors may need to be addressed.

Among those factors to be considered are sleep, exercise and nutrition. For example, extremes of sleep promote illness, impaired exercise and improper nutrition. Extremes of exercise promote injury, chronic fatigue and susceptibility to illness. Extremes of nutrition cause weight gain or loss, which, in turn, affect multiple systems and so on.

T̴ʜᴇ Accordion Reserve© *Hʏᴘᴏᴛʜᴇsɪs*

Every environmental factor and human energy field has the potential to contribute to the cause and effect of an illness.

At present, it is extremely expensive and difficult to design experiments that account for an infinite number of triggers (the Accordion Handles), complex symptoms and signs (movement of the Accordion Bellows) and diversity of treatments (the Handles). Yet, it has been done on a limited basis. Dr. Rea reported details in studies documenting environmentally triggered thrombophlebitis, vasculitis and cardiac disease.[3]

However, in studies on atherosclerotic heart disease, experiments control for six to ten variables – age, gender, weight, blood pressure, cholesterol, triglycerides, exercise, diabetes, episodes of chest pain, family history, previous heart attacks, medication dosage and adverse effects.

Results do not always agree with predictions: "statin" drugs lower cholesterol in occlusive coronary artery disease, but improvement is unrelated to an increase in diameter of blocked blood vessels. Instead, current thinking is that reversal of inflammation is the mechanism for improvement. With the Accordion Reserve© hypothesis other variables should be included: daily nutrition, vitamins, minerals, emotional stress, hormones, other chemical mediators, exposures to pollutants, infections, weather, radiation, electromagnetic fields, etc. More comprehensively defined variables could have changed the conclusions of Muntwyler et al. in observing that vitamin supplementation did not affect cardiovascular outcomes.[4]

Another example of incomplete data is recent studies[5,6,7] reporting that infants who suck a pacifier are more prone to ear infections. An older study[8] identified increased N-nitrosamines in infants who had sucked on baby-bottle nipples and pacifiers. The first 3 did not assess whether infants sucking on a pacifier were being exposed to latex, silicone or other chemicals. These substances might contribute to some infants' impaired immunity, which, in turn, could predispose them to more frequent infections.

Additional factors (how chemical processes in the liver are working, how different lengths of the intestines are absorbing nutrients) may also influence your Accordion Reserve© at any moment. Thus, the number of variables that affect your RESERVE is theoretically limitless. So, too, is the size of your Accordion Reserve©.

THINKING OUTSIDE THE BLACK BOX

♫♫♫♫♫

I mentioned in Chapter 3 that the Accordion Reserve© is a powerful reminder of my family legacy. Once the Accordion model became apparent to Natalie and me, we began to find ways to validate our hypothesis. One idea I had was to create a multidimensional stress test to maximally challenge an individual. I then focused on stress tests that are already in use.

Stress tests are used routinely to challenge patients. These are categorized into those same factors on the Energy Handle of the Accordion:

* Exercise stress tests
* Sleep-deprived EEG, polysomnograms (sleep stressor)
* Glucose-tolerance test, water fasts (nutritional stressor)
* Timed-response stress tests to test the heart (emotional stressor)

Autonomic Stress Tests The ANSAR®[9] technology evaluates the ANS by challenging the PSNS by a deep breathing challenge, the SNS by a Valsalva challenge and both branches by a stand challenge. I realized that these "stress tests" were compatible with the movement of the Accordion – the functional dynamic mode described above.

MULTIPLE SYSTEM INVOLVEMENT

I recognized that patients with ANS abnormalities on ANSAR® testing also had multiple system involvement. In these patients, I had no definite priority to the order of treatment other than to treat the most affected system first (as recognized by symptoms or degree of potential mortality). Occasionally, I treated the ANS first. In "ANS-first patients," it appeared that additional treatments of subsequent systems resulted in fewer side effects compared to "other organ system treated first."

ANS as Controller Thus, I hypothesized that the ANS has a priority relative to all other organ systems, serving them as an umbrella and controller. Inherently, this hypothesis makes sense since PSNS regulates primary activity of all organs systems.

I then thought of the ANS as a protective umbrella or roof. Because PSNS and SNS meet in the brain stem at the nucleus solitarius, I imagined the ANS at the apex connected to 2 sides of a triangle. The Accordion then fit in as the base of that triangle (**Figure PC-4**).

Accordion as Musculoskeletal System I recognized that the Accordion's Environmental Handle is a physical representation, and the Energy Handle is a mental representation (see also these referenced connections of the chakras in Chapter 11). Then I associated the "musculoskeletal system" (MS) with the Environmental/Physical

Handle and the "emotional system" (ES) with the Energy Handle.

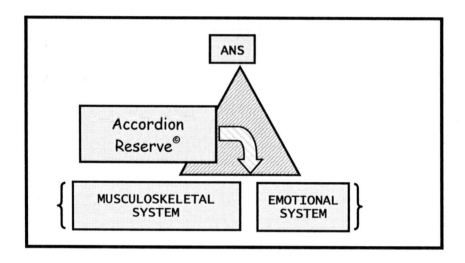

Figure PC-4. **Accordion Reserve**© and ANS. The ANS is the apex of the triangle, and the Accordion is its base. MS is on the Environmental Handle; ES is on the Energy Handle.

As other physicians have observed, I recognized during exams that patients with ANS abnormalities usually had balance disturbances when challenged with their eyes closed. Many of these individuals also had relatively inflexible musculoskeletal systems.

ANS AND FLEXIBILITY

I hypothesized that:
* More flexible ANS ⇒ more flexible MS and ES.
* More rigid ANS ⇒ more rigid MS and ES.
* In other words, the body functions more effectively when the ANS is flexible.

♫♫♫♫♫

Flexibility of MS - Less Injury, More Rapid Healing
The following analogies simplify the concept of potential for injury
and healing:
* When muscles, ligaments and tendons are flexible, injury
  is less likely.
* Inflexibility of muscles and supporting structures promotes potential for injury.
* Unexpected injuries will more likely heal faster if ANS
  and MS are flexible.

Skill Performance is more precise when MS is more flexible. Example:
* A soccer player controls the ball by "trapping" it. If he is
  flexible, he functions like a cushion when he positions
  himself to receive the ball against his body, causing the
  ball to drop near him.
* The reverse is also true. An inflexible player performs
  like a stone statue, and the ball bounds far from the
  player.

ANS Flexibility and Any Organ System Apply the same
thinking to any other organ system. Better ANS function (i.e. it is
more flexible) results in improved organ system and organ function.
In optimal health, the ANS would be finely tuned and infinitely
flexible. The ANS would direct an appropriate response of the organ
or organ system as required. The ANS would respond quickly and
precisely to the stress, and ideally, no excess expenditure of energy
would be required. In many situations, optimal health would not even
require additional input of the ANS.

MULTIPLE SYSTEMS

A triangle can be drawn to represent each organ system, since
the ANS interacts with and controls each of them.

Each of the following **Figures PC-5, PC-6 and PC-7** represent a progression in the development of the working model.

ANS AND THE HYPOTHALAMIC-PITUITARY AXIS

The ANS has multiple connections throughout the brain. Broadly speaking the deeper controlling structures of the brain are called the hypothalamic-pituitary axis (HPA). These structures control appetite, temperature, hormones and many more functions. Most importantly, the ANS integrates and relates to the HPA as in **Figure PC-5.**

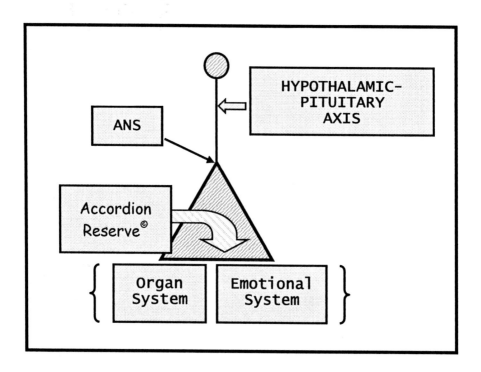

Figure PC-5. ANS and Hypothalamic-Pituitary Axis. The connections between these brain structures regulate complex body functions.

Active Organ System Now look at the figure below and observe that the triangle can spin on the pole of the HPA, just like a reflecting sphere in a concert hall. **Figure PC-6** illustrates this globe effect.

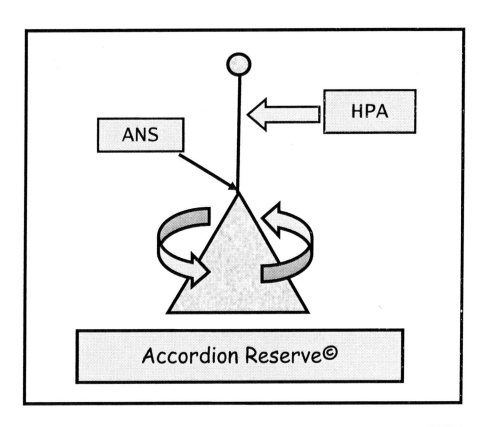

Figure PC-6. Spinning the **Accordion Reserve**[©] Triangle on the HPA Creates a Global Effect.

HPA, ANS AND MULTIPLE ORGANS

Finally, consider multiple organ systems functioning at the same time, all spinning, interacting with the ANS and the HPA. Since the Accordion Reserve© will be functioning differently for each system, imagine multiple dimples or bumps on the surface of a globe, each system changing as it spins on the HPA.

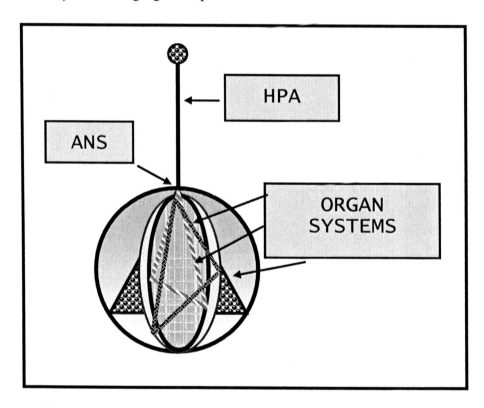

Figure PC-7. Three Organ Systems Spinning on HPA, Creating Global Effect. The sphere functions like a balloon, expanding and collapsing. Each organ system functions with its own Accordion.

The **Accordion Reserve**© is a working model to encourage researchers to explore the multitude of variables that promote health and illness.

As a hypothesis it is proposed that energy inputs are stresses that may be negative or positive. Environmental factors and energy factors are stressors that stimulate a response by the individual. In a stable health system, the stress may not require ANS attention. More stressful triggers will provoke an ANS response.

In a healthy individual (Environmental Health) the ANS responds in a flexible manner to guide and direct each organ system to respond by returning the individual to his prior state of health. A desirable stress results in an ANS response, accumulating energy, resulting in improved ANS balance.

Sustained negative (undesirable) stresses result in SNS overactivity, a gradually failing PSNS and a less flexible ANS. This dynamic is represented by a collapsing Accordion and is described as Environmentally Triggered Illness.

In the hypothesis, the dynamic of multiple organ system involvement is represented by a globe, over the span of time spinning on the hypothalamic-pituitary axis (HPA), simultaneously pulsing, as influenced by the movement of the Accordion for each organ system.

The hypothesis suggests that as more organ systems become involved, it is increasingly likely that autonomic dysfunction is present. Therefore, during evaluation, early detection of ANS dysfunction prior to overt symptoms is strongly encouraged. Hidden stressors such as impaired communication pathways may be, in effect, jeopardizing health.

Using the descriptive Accordion as a basis for illness detection and treatment, health care providers should investigate environmental factor contributions to illness. They can then initiate appropriate corrective therapies that address mechanisms pertinent to the identified abnormalities, thus contributing to restoration of ANS balance.

As a working model, the hypothesis predicts that there is an energetic basis for maintaining and restoring Environmental Health. The sources for energy management are balanced sleep, exercise, nutrition, relationships and a belief system.

The health care traditions of many cultures are assimilated in the model. This concept encourages a unity of thinking rather than confrontation and adversity.

The basis for healing is dependent on establishing a balanced ANS. This balance is predicated on relaxed, conditioned PSNS breathing, recognizing **Body Awareness**, discovering and discarding hidden negative energy stressors and promoting **Spiritual Healing**. The result of these efforts is a unified **Mind/body/soul/spirit**.

Researchers: Please critically review and test **the Accordion Reserve**© model and hypothesis. We encourage open discussion, study and learning. Critique, confirm, revise and expand. In this pursuit, we all will profit.

SUMMARY

1) The ANS directs and controls every organ system, represented by a triangle relationship. The SNS and PSNS relate to each other directly in the brain stem.

2) The ANS relates to higher portions of the brain through a stalk called the HPA.

3) Descriptively, each organ triangle is suspended from the pole of the HPA.

4) Each organ triangle spins on the pole. The effect is to create a sphere, spinning on the pole.

5) Representing an organ system, the base of each triangle continuously moves according to the function of its own Accordion.

6) Environmental Health is represented by an enlarged spinning sphere (like a balloon), expanding and collapsing, like active, breathing lungs and chest wall.

7) Dimples in the surface of the sphere represent degrees of illness. The dimples suggest a relatively collapsed Accordion for a given organ system.

8) Environmentally Triggered Illness and chronic diseases are represented by a small sphere, with variable sized depressions. These craters result from poorly performing **Accordion Reserves**© of many organ systems.

9) Environmental Health is represented by a flexible, expanded sphere, each organ system responding quickly with only small adjustments required as needed to restore the body to health.

---

[1]Randolph TG. 1962. *Human Ecology and Susceptibility to the Chemical Environment.* Charles C Thomas, Publisher, Springfield, IL. Any new student of Environmental Medicine is encouraged to read this groundbreaking book.
[2] Ashford N, Miller CS. 1997. *Chemical Exposures. Low Levels and High Stakes.* 2nd Edition. Van Nostrand Publishers, New York.
[3] Rea WJ. 1977. *Ann. Allergy* 37:101. *Ann. Allergy* 38:245, and *Ann. Allergy* 40:243.
[4] Muntwyler J, Hennekens CH, Manson JE, Buring JE, Gaziano JM. 2002.Vitamin supplement use in a low-risk population of US male physicians and subsequent cardiovascular mortality. *Arch Int Med* 162:1472-76.
[5] Ford-Jones EL, et al. 2002. Microbiologic findings and risk factors for antimicrobial resistance at myringotomy for tympanostomy tube placement – a prospective study of 601 children in Toronto. *Intl J Ped Oto* 66:227-42.
[6] Jackson JM, Mourino AP. 1999. Pacifier use and otitis media in infants twelve months of age or younger. *Pediatric Dentistry* 21:255-60.
[7] Hanafin S, Griffiths P. 2002. Does pacifier use cause ear infections in young children? *British Jl of Community Nursing* 7:206, 208-11.
[8] Westin JB. 1990. Ingestion of carcinogenic N-nitrosamines by infants and children. *Arch Env Health* 45:359-63.
[9] ANSAR Inc. 240 South Eighth St Philadelphia, PA 19107, 888-883-7804, 215-922-6088.

PART IX

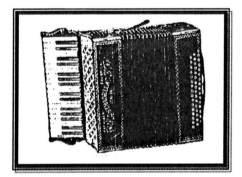

APPENDIX

APPENDIX A FOOD FAMILIES:
List 1 Alphabetical

A

81	abalone
80	absinthe
41	acacia (gum)
46	acerola
79	acorn squash
1	agar agar
12	agave
98	albacore
41	alfalfa
1	Algae Family
63	allspice
40b	almond
11	*Aloe vera*
54	althea root
30	amaranth
12	Amaryllis Family
94	amberjack
86	American eel
117	*Amphibians*
85	anchovy
65	angelica
65	anise
38	annatto
136	antelope
40a	apple
73	apple mint
40b	apricot
47	arrowroot, Brazilian (tapioca)
9	arrowroot *(Colocasia)*
17	arrowroot, East Indian *(Curcuma)*
19	Arrowroot Family
13	arrowroot, Figi *(Tacca)*
4	arrowroot, Florida *(Zamia)*
19	arrowroot *(Maranta* starch)
16	arrowroot *(Musa)*
18	arrowroot, Queensland
80	artichoke flour
80	artichoke (globe)
80	artichoke, Jerusalem
9	Arum Family
11	asparagus
2	*Aspergillus*
34	avocado
41	azuki beans

B

2	baker's yeast
6	bamboo shoots
16	banana
16	Banana Family
46	Barbados cherry
6	barley
73	basil
114	bass (black)
113	bass (yellow)
53	basswood
34	bay leaf
41	bean
132	bear
66	bearberry
24	Beech Family
137	beef
28	beet
74	bell pepper
73	bergamot
121	birds
23	Birch Family
38	Bixa Family
114	black bass
40c	blackberry
41	black beans
41	black-eyed peas
21	black pepper
80	black salsify

22	black walnut	41	carob
66	blueberry	111	carp
93	bluefish	29	Carpetweed Family
80	boneset	1	carageen
98	bonito	65	carrot
71	Boston marrow	65	Carrot Family
71	borage	79	casaba melon
79	Borage Family	79	caserta squash
40c	boysenberry	48	cashew
137	Bovine Family	48	Cashew Family
6	bran	47	cassava
52	brandy	34	cassia bark
47	Brazilian arrowroot	47	castor oil
62	Brazil nut	112	catfish, lake
25	breadfruit	112	Catfish Family, lake
2	brewer's yeast	88	catfish (ocean)
36	broccoli	88	Catfish Family, sea
36	Brussels sprouts	73	catnip
27	buckwheat	36	cauliflower
27	Buckwheat Family	104	caviar
137	buffalo/bison	74	cayenne pepper
6	bulgur	65	celeriac
80	burdock root	65	celery
40	burnet	80	celtuce
31	Buttercup Family	9	ceriman
79	buttercup squash	80	chamomile
101	butterfish	52	champagne
22	butternut	28	chard
79	butternut squash	79	chayote
		32	cherimoya
	C	40b	cherry
		65	chervil
36	cabbage	24	chestnut
55	cacao	73	chia seed
60	Cactus Family	124	chicken
70	camote	41	chickpea
6	cane sugar	67	chicle
18	Canna Family	80	chicory
36	canola (rapeseed)	74	chili pepper
79	cantaloupe	36	Chinese cabbage
37	caper	56	Chinese gooseberry
37	Caper Family	14	Chinese potato
74	*Capsicum*	79	Chinese preserving melon
42	carambola	7	Chinese water chestnut
65	caraway seed	24	chinquapin
17	cardamom	11	chives
80	cardoon	55	chocolate
135	caribou		

111	chub
7	chufa
40a	cider
34	cinnamon
1	citric acid
45	citron
6	citronella
45	Citrus Family
81	clam
73	clary
63	clove
41	clover
55	cocoa
55	cocoa butter
8	coconut
79	cocozelle
87	Codfish Family
87	cod (scrod)
76	coffee
55	cola nut
36	collards
80	coltsfoot
36	colza shoots
71	comfrey
80	Composite Family
5	Conifer Family
65	coriander
6	corn
124	cornish hen
78	corn-salad
80	costmary
54	cottonseed oil
41	coumarin
36	couve tronchuda
41	cowpea
82	crab
40a	crabapple
66	cranberry
114	crappie
82	crayfish
52	cream of tartar
79	Crenshaw melon
96	croaker
79	crookneck squash
79	cucumber
65	cumin
36	curly cress

39	currant
79	cushaw squash
87	cusk
32	custard-apple
32	Custard-Apple Family
4	Cycad Family

D

103	dab
80	dandelion
9	dasheen
8	date
8	date sugar
135	deer
40c	dewberry
65	dill
56	Dillenia Family
73	dittany
95	dolphin
122	dove
52	dried "currant"
96	drum (saltwater)
116	drum (freshwater)
121	duck
1	dulse

E

17	East Indian arrowroot
68	Ebony Family
124	egg, chicken
121	egg, duck
121	egg, goose
121	egg, guinea fowl
126	egg, turkey
74	eggplant
77	elderberry
135	elk
80	endive
22	Eaglish walnut
80	escarole
63	eucalyptus

F

41	fava bean
65	fennel

5	juniper

K

68	kaki
36	kale
1	kelp
41	kidney bean
56	kiwi berry
36	kohlrabi
45	kumquat

L

137	lamb
28	lamb's-quarters
34	Laurel Family
73	lavender
41	lecithin
11	leek
41	Legume Family
45	lemon
73	lemon balm
6	lemon grass
72	lemon verbena
41	Lentil
80	lettuce
41	licorice
11	Lily Family
41	lima bean
45	lime
53	linden
53	Linden Family
44	linseed
51	litchi
82	lobster
40c	loganberry
79	loofah
40a	loquat
65	lovage
79	Luffa
51	lychee

M

26	macadamia
33	mace
98	mackerel

76	Madder Family
95	mahi mahi
9	malanga
54	Mallow Family
46	Malpighia Family
6	malt
6	maltose
127	mammals
48	mango
50	Maple Family
50	maple products
19	*Maranta* starch
73	marjoram
99	marlin
49	maté
84	menhaden
12	mescal
6	millet
137	milk, cow's, goat's, sheep's
137	milk products
6	milo
73	Mint Family
6	molasses
2	mold
135	moose
2	morel
70	Morning-Glory Family
25	mulberry
25	Mulberry Family
89	mullet
41	mung bean
45	murcot
52	muscadine
2	mushroom
109	muskellunge
79	muskmelon
36	Mustard Family
36	mustard greens
36	mustard seed/powder
137	mutton
63	Myrtle Family

N

14	ñame
43	nasturtium
43	Nasturtium Family
41	navy bean

40b	nectarine	40a	pear
29	New Zealand spinach	22	pecan
97	northern scup	40a	pectin
33	nutmeg	75	Pedalium Family
33	Nutmeg Family	73	pennyroyal
2	nutritional yeast	74	pepino
		74	pepper, bell (sweet)
	O	74	pepper, cayenne
		74	pepper, chili
6	oat	74	pepper, sweet
6	oatmeal	21	Pepper Family
88	ocean catfish	21	peppercorn
102	ocean perch	73	peppermint
23	oil of birch	102	perch (ocean)
54	okra	113	perch (white)
69	olive	115	perch (yellow)
69	Olive Family	79	Persian melon
11	onion	68	persimmon
128	opossum	124	pheasant
45	orange	109	pickerel
28	Orchid Family	122	pigeon (squab)
73	oregano	30	pigweed
15	orris root	109	pike
42	oxalis	84	pilchard (sardine)
42	Oxalis Family	63	*Pimenta*
81	oyster	74	pimiento
80	oyster plant	10	pineapple
		10	Pineapple Family
	P	5	pine nut
		41	pinto beans
8	palm cabbage	21	*Piper*
8	Palm Family	48	pistachio
59	papaya	103	plaice
59	Papaya Family	16	plantain
74	paprika	40b	plum
62	paradise nut	9	poi
65	parsley	48	poison ivy
65	parsnip	87	pollack
123	partridge	61	pomegranate
58	Passion Flower Family	61	Pomegranate Family
58	passion fruit	94	pompano
6	patent flour	6	popcorn
79	pattypan squash	35	Poppy Family
32	pawpaw	35	poppy seed
41	pea, green	97	porgy
40b	peach	134	pork
124	peafowl	74	potato
41	peanut		

74	Potato Family	54	roselle
82	prawn	73	rosemary
79	preserving melon	45	Rue Family
60	prickly pear	123	ruffed grouse
26	Protea Family	36	rutabaga
40b	prune	6	rye
2	puffball		
12	pulque		**S**
45	pummelo		
79	pumpkin	80	safflower oil
79	pumpkin seed	15	saffron
114	pumpkinseed (sunfish)	73	sage
30	purslane	8	sago starch
30	Purslane Family	99	sailfish
80	pyrethrum	106	salmon species
		80	salsify
	Q	80	santolina
		67	Sapodilla Family
124	quail	62	Sapucaya Family
18	Queensland arrowroot	62	sapucaya nut
26	Queensland nut	84	sardine (pilchard)
40	quince	11	sarsaparilla
28	quinoa	34	sassafras
		115	sauger (perch)
	R	73	savory
		39	Saxifrage Family
129	rabbit	81	scallop
36	radish	80	scolymus
52	raisin	80	scorzonera
11	ramp	91	Sea Bass Family
36	rapeseed	88	Sea Catfish Family
40c	raspberry	27	sea grape
119	rattlesnake	84	sea herring
41	red clover	96	sea trout
138	red snapper	1	seaweed
138	Red Snapper Family	7	Sedge Family
135	reindeer	6	semolina
118	Reptiles	41	senna
139	Requien Family	75	sesame
27	rhubarb	105	shad
6	rice	11	shallot
6	rice syrup	139	shark
137	Rocky Mountain sheep	3	shavegrass
105	roe	137	sheep
80	romaine	82	shrimp
40	Rose Family	96	silver perch
102	rosefish	90	silverside
40a	rosehips	98	skipjack

40b	sloe
108	smelt
81	snail
138	Snapper Family
138	snapper
51	Soapberry Family
11	soap plant
103	sole
6	sorghum
27	sorrel
80	southerwood
41	soybean
41	soy products
73	spearmint
6	spelt
28	spinach
96	spot
7	spotted sea trout
47	Spurge Family
79	squash
81	squid
130	squirrel
55	Sterculia Family
80	stevia rebaudiana
40c	strawberry
41	string bean
104	sturgeon
110	sucker
28	sugar beet
6	sugar cane
73	summer savory
114	sunfish
80	sunflower seed
36	swede
65	sweet cicely
6	sweet corn
74	sweet pepper
70	sweet potato
70	sweet potato flour
100	swordfish

T

13	Tacca Family
75	tahini
41	tamarind
28	tampala
45	tangelo

45	tangerine
80	tansy
47	tapioca
9	taro
80	tarragon
57	tea
57	Tea Family
6	teff
12	tequila
120	terrapin
73	thyme
92	tilefish
74	tobacco
41	tofu
74	tomatillo
74	tomato
41	tonka bean
74	tree tomato
6	triticale
106	trout species
2	truffle
98	tuna
79	turban squash
103	turbot
126	turkey
17	turmeric
36	turnip
120	turtle species

U

36	upland cress

V

78	Valerian Family
20	vanilla
137	veal
79	vegetable spaghetti
135	venison
72	Verbena Family
40a	vinegar (apple cider)

W

115	walleye
22	Walnut Family
7	water chestnut, Chinese

36	watercress
79	watermelon
96	weakfish
131	whale
6	wheat
6	wheat germ
90	whitebait
107	whitefish
21	white pepper
113	white perch
87	whiting
6	wild rice
40c	wineberry
52	wine vinegar
23	wintergreen
73	winter savory
80	witloof chicory
76	woodruff
80	wormwood

Y

14	yam
14	Yam Family
14	yampi
80	yarrow
9	yautia
2	yeast
113	yellow bass
94	yellow jack
115	yellow perch
79	yellow squash
49	yerba maté
40c	youngberry
47	yuca
11	yucca

Z

4	*Zamia*
79	zucchini

APPENDIX B FOOD FAMILIES:
List II Numerical

PLANT

1 - Algae Family
    agar agar
    carrageen (Irish moss)
  * dulse
    kelp (seaweed)

2 - Fungi Family
    baker's yeast
    brewer's or nutritional
    yeast
    citric acid *(Aspergillus)*
    mold (in certain cheeses)
    morel
    mushroom
    puffball
    truffle

3- Horsetail Family,
    Equisetaceae
  * shavegrass (horsetail)

4 - Cycad Family, *Cycadaceae*
    Florida arrowroot *(Zamia)*

5 - Conifer Family, *Coniferae*
  * jumper (gin)
    pine nut (pinon, pinyon)

6- Grass Family, *Graminaea*
    bamboo shoots
    barley
      malt
      maltose
    corn (mature)
      corn meal
      cornoil
      cornstarch

      corn sugar
      hominy grits
      popcorn
    lemon grass
      citronella
    millet
    milo
    oat
      oatmeal
    rice
      rice flour
      rice syrup
    rye
      rye flour
    sorghum grain
      syrup
    spelt
    sugar cane
      cane sugar
      molasses
    teff
    triticale
    wheat
      bran
      bulgur
      flour
      gluten
      graham
      patent
      semolina
      whole wheat
      wheat germ
    wild rice

7 - Sedge Family, *Cyperaceae*
    Chinese water chestnut
    chufa (groundnut)

* One or more plant parts (leaf, root, seed, etc.) used as beverage.

8 -   Palm Family, *Palmacaeae*
  coconut
   coconut meal
   coconut oil
  date
   date sugar
  palm cabbage
  sago starch *(Metroxylon)*

9 -   Arum Family, *Araceae*
  ceriman *(Monstera)*
  dasheen *(Colocasia)*
   arrowroot
  malanga *(Xanthosoma)*
  taro *(Colocasia)*
   arrowroot
   poi
  yautia *(Xanthosoma)*

10 - Pineapple Family,
  Bromeliaceae
  pineapple

11 - Lily Family, *Lillaceae*
  Aloe vera
  asparagus
  chives
  garlic
  leek
  onion
  ramp
 * sarsaparilla
  shallot
  yucca (soap plant)

12 - Amaryllis Family,
  Amaryllidaceae
  agave
   mescal
   pulque
   tequila

13-   Tacca Family, *Taccaceae*
  Fiji arrowroot *(Tacca)*

14 - Yam Family, *Dioscoreaceae*
  Chinese potato (yam)
  ñame (yampi)

15 - Iris Family, *Iridaceae*
  orris root (scant)
  saffron (Crocus)

16 - Banana Family, *Muscaeae*
  arrowroot *(Musa)*
  banana
  plantain

17 - Ginger Family,
  Zingiberaceae
  cardamom
  East Indian arrowroot
  (Curcuma)
  ginger
  tumeric

18 - Canna Family, *Cannaceae*
  Queensland arrowroot

19 - Arrowroot Family,
  Marantaceae
  arrowroot *(Maranta starch)*

20 - Orchid Family, *Orchidaceae*
  vanilla

21 - Pepper Family, *Piperaceae*
  peppercorn *(Piper)*
   black pepper
   white pepper

22 - Walnut Family,
  Juglandaceae
  black walnut
  butternut
  English walnut
  heartnut
  hickory nut
  pecan

23 - Birch Family, *Betulaceae*
  filbert (hazelnut)

oil of birch
(wintergreen)
(some wintergreen flavor is
methyl salicylate)

24 - Beech Family, *Fagaceae*
chestnut
chinquapin

25 - Mulberry Family, *Moraceae*
breadfruit
fig
  * hop
mulberry

26- Protea Family, *Proteaceae*
macademia
(Queensland nut)

27 - Buckwheat Family,
Polygonaceae
buckwheat
garden sorrel
rhubarb
sea grape

28 - Goosefoot Family,
Chenopodiaceae
beet
lamb's quarters
quinoa
spinach
sugar beet
Swiss chard
tampala

29 - Carpetweed Family,
Aizoaceae
New Zealand spinach

30 - Purslane Family,
Portulacaceae
amaranth
pigweed (purslane)

31 - Buttercup Family,
Ranunculaceae

  * golden seal

32 - Custard-Apple Family
Annonaceae
cherimoya
custard-apple
papaw (paw-paw)

33 - Nutmeg Family,
Myristicaceae
nutmeg
mace

34 - Laurel Family, *Lauraceae*
avocado
bay leaf
cassia bark
cinnamon
  * sassafras
file (powder)

35 - Poppy Family,
Papaveraceae
poppyseed

36 - Mustard Family, *Cruciferae*
broccoli
Brussels sprouts
cabbage
canola oil
cardoon
cauliflower
Chinese cabbage
collards
colza shoots
couve tronshuda
curley cress
daicon
horseradish
kale
kohlrabi
mustard greens
   mustard seed/powder
radish
rapeseed (oil)
rutabaga (swede)
turnip
   turnip greens

upland cress
watercress

37 - Caper Family,
Capparidaceae
caper

38 - Bixa Family, *Bixaceae*
annatto
(natural yellow dye)

39 - Saxifrage Family,
Saxifragaceae
currant
gooseberry

40 - Rose Family, *Rosaceae*
a. pomes
apple
crabapple
loquat
pear
pectin
quince
rosehips
b. stone fruits
almond
apricot
cherry
nectarine
peach
plum (prune)
sloe
c. berries
blackberry
boysenberry
dewberry
loganberry
raspberry
black raspberry
purple raspberry
strawberry
wineberry
d. herb
burnet
(cucumber flavor)

41 - Legume Family,
Leguminoseae
alfalfa (sprouts)
anasazi beans
black beans
black-eyed peas (cowpea)
carob
carob syrup
fava beans
fenugreek
garbanzo beans (chickpea)
green beans (string)
gum acacia
jicama
kidney beans
kudzu
lentil
licorice
lima beans
mung beans (sprouts)
navy beans
pea
peanut
peanut oil
red clover
senna
soy bean
lecithin
soy flour
soy grits
soy milk
soy oil
tamarind
tonka bean
coumarin

42 - Oxalis Family, *Oxalidaceae*
carambola
oxalis

43 - Nasturtium Family,
Tropaeoloceae
nasturtium

44 - Flax Family, *Linaceae*
flaxseed
linseed oil

45 - Rue (Citrus) Family,
Ruaceae
   citron
   grapefruit
   kumquat
   lemon
   lime
   murcot
   orange
   pummelo
   tangelo
   tangerine

46 - Malpighia Family,
Malpighiaceae
   acerola (Barbados cherry)

47 - Spurge Family,
Euphorbiaceae
   cassava or yuca *(Manihot)*
     cassava meal *(manioc)*
     tapioca
     (Brazilian arrowroot)
   castor bean
     castor oil

48 - Cashew Family,
Anacardiaceae
   cashew
   mango
   pistachio

49 - Holly Family, *Aquifoliaceae*
   maté (yerba maté)

50 - Maple Family, *Aceraceae*
   maple sugar
   maple syrup

51 - Soapberry Family,
Sapindaceae
   litchi (lychee)

52 - Grape Family, *Vitaceae*
   grape
     brandy
     champagne
     cream of tartar
     dried "currant"
     muscadine
     raisin
     wine
     wine vinegar

53 - Linden Family, *Tiliceae*
*   basswood (linden)

54 - Mallow Family, *Malvaceae*
*   althea root
   cottonseed oil
*   hibiscus (roselle)
   okra

55 - Sterculia Family,
Sterculiaceae
   chocolate (cacao)
*   cocoa
     cocoa butter
   cola nut

56 - Dillenia Family,
Dilleniacece
   Chinese gooseberry (kiwi)

57 - Tea Family, *Theaceae*
*   tea

58 - Passion Flower Family,
Passifloraceae
   granadilla
     (passion fruit)

59 - Papaya Family, *Caricaceae*
   papaya

60 - Cactus Family, *Cactaceae*
   prickly pear

61 - Pomegranate Family,
Puniceae
   grenadine
   pomegranate

62 - Sapucaya Family,
 Lecythidaceae
   Brazil nut
   sapucaya nut
     (paradise nut)

63 - Myrtle Family, *Myrtaceae*
   allspice *(Pimenta)*
   clove
 * eucalyptus
   guava

64 - Ginseng Family, *Araliaceae*
 * American ginseng
 * Chinese ginseng

65 - Carrot Family, *Umbelliferae*
   angelica
   anise
   caraway
   carrot
   celeriac (celery root)
   celery
 * celery seed and leaf
   chervil
   coriander
   cumin
   dill
     dill seed
   fennel
     finocchio
     Florence fennel
 * gotu kola
 * lovage
 * parsley
   parsnip
   sweet cecily

66 - Heath Family, *Ericaceae*
 * bearberry
 * blueberry
   cranberry
 * huckleberry

67 - Sapodilla Family,
 Sapotaceae
   chicle (chewing gum)

68 - Ebony Family, *Ebonaceae*
   American persimmon
   kaki (Japanese persimmon)

69 - Olive Family, *Oleaceae*
   olive (green olive)
   olive oil

70 - Morning Glory Family,
 Concolculacea
   camote
   sweet potato

71 - Borage Family, *Boraginceae*
   borage (oil)
 * comfrey leaf and root

72 - Verbena Family,
 Verbenaceae
 * lemon verbena

73 - Mint Family (Herbs),
 Labiatae
   apple mint
   basil
   bergamot
 * catnip
 * chia seed
   clary
 * dittany
 * horehound
 * hyssop
   lavender
   lemon balm
   marjoram
   oregano
 * pennyroyal
 * peppermint
   rosemary
   sage
 * spearmint
   summer savory
   thyme
   winter savory

74 - Potato Family, *Solanaceae*
   eggplant

ground cherry
pepino (melon pear)
pepper *(Capsicum)*
  bell, sweet
  cayenne
  chili pepper
  green pepper
  hot pepper
  paprika
pimiento
potato
tobacco
tomatillo
tomato
tree tomato

75 - Pedalium Family,
  Pedaliceae
  sesame seed
    sesame oil
      tahini

76 - Madder Family, *Rubiceae*
 * coffee
  woodruff

77 - Honeysuckle Family,
  Caprifoliaceae
  elderberry

78 - Valerian Family,
  Valerianceae
  corn salad (fetticus)

79 - Gourd Family,
  Cucurbitaceae
  chayote
  Chinese reserving melon
  cucumber
  gherkin
  melons
    cantaloupe
    casaba
    crenshaw
    honeydew
    Persionmelon

muskmelon
watermelon
pumpkin
  pumpkin seed
squashes
  acorn
  buttercup
  butternut
  Boston marrow
  caserta
  cocozelle
  crookneck
  cushaw
  golden nugget
  Hubbard varieties
  patty pan
  straightneck
  turban
  vegetable spaghetti
  yellow
  zucchini

80 - Composite Family,
  Compositae
 * boneset
 * burdock root
  cardoon
 * chamomile
 * chicory
  coltsfoot
  costmary
  dandelion
  endive
  escarole
  globe artichoke
 * goldenrod
 * Jerusalem artichoke
    artichoke flour
  lettuce
    Boston Bibb
    celtuce
    iceberg
    leaf
    romaine
  pyrethrum (Not Edible)
  safflower oil
  salsify (oyster plant)
  santolina (herb)

scolymus
  (Spanish oyster plant)
scorzonera (black salsify)
southernwood
stevia rebaudiana
sunflower seed
  sunflower oil
tansy (herb)
tarragon
witloof chicory
  (French endive)
wormwood (absinthe)
* yarrow

ANIMAL

81 - SEAFOOD

81 - <u>Mollusks</u>
  abalone
  clam
  cockle
  mussel
  Moyster
  scallop
  snail
  squid

82 - <u>Crustaceans</u>
  crab
  crayfish
  lobster
  prawn
  shrimp

83- <u>FISHES (SALTWATER)</u>

84 - Herring Family
  menhaden
  pilchard (sardine)
  sea herring

85 - Anchovy Family
  anchovy

86 - Eel Family
  American eel

87- Codfish Family
  cod (scrod)
  cusk
  haddock
  hake
  pollack
  whiting

88- Sea Catfish Family
  ocean catfish

89 - Mullet Family
  mullet

90 - Silverside Family
  silverside (whitebait)

91- Seabass Family
  grouper
  sea bass

92 - Tilefish Family
  tilefish

93- Bluefish Family
  bluefish

94 - Jack Family
  amberjack
  pompano
  yellow jack

95 - Dolphin Family
  dolphin

96 - Croaker Family
  croaker
  drum
  sea trout
  silver perch
  spot
  weakfish (spotted sea
  trout)

97 - Porgy Family
  northern scup (porgy)

98 - Mackerel Family
   albacore
   bonito
   mackerel
   skipjack
   tuna

99 - Marlin Family
   marlin
   sailfish

100 - Swordfish Family
   swordfish

101 - Harvestfish Family
   butterfish
   harvestflsh

102 - Scorpionfish Family
   rosefish (ocean perch)

103A - Flounder Family
   dab
   flounder
   halibut
   plaice
   sole
   turbot

103B - Snapper Family
   red snapper

103C - Requien Family
   shark

104 - **FISHES (FRESHWATER)**

104 - Sturgeon Family
   sturgeon (caviar)

105 - Herring Family
   shad (roe)

106 - Salmon Family
   salmon species
   trout species

107 - Whitefish Family
   whitefish

108 - Smelt Family
   smelt

109 - Pike Family
   muskellunge
   pickerel
   pike

110 - Sucker Family
   buffalofish
   sucker

111- Minnow Family
   carp
   chub

112 - Catfish Family
   lake catfish species

113 - Bass Family
   white perch
   yellow bass

114 - Sunfish Family
   black bass species
   crappie
   sunfish species
   pumpkinseed

115 - Perch Family
   sauger
   walleye
   yellow perch

116 - Croaker Family
   freshwater drum

117 - **AMPHIBIANS**

117 - Frog Family
   frog (frog legs)

118 - <u>REPTILES</u>

119 - Snake Family
    rattlesnake

120 - Turtle Family
    terpapin
    turtle species

121 - <u>BIRDS</u>

121 - Duck Family
    duck
      duck eggs
    goose
      goose eggs

122 - Dove Family
    dove
    pigeon (squab)

123 - Grouse Family
    ruffed grouse
    (partridge)

124 - Pheasant Family
    chicken
      chicken eggs
    cornish hen
    peafowl
    pheasant
    quail

125 - Guinea Fowl Family
    guinea fowl
      guinea fowl eggs

126 - Turkey Family
    turkey
      turkey eggs

127 - <u>MAMMALS</u>

128 - Opossum Family
    opossum

129 - Hare Family
    rabbit

130 - Squirrel Family
    squirrel

131 - Whale Family
    whale

132 - Bear Family
    bear

133 - Horse Family
    horse

134 - Swine Family
    hog (pork)
      bacon
      ham
      lard
      pork gelatin
      sausage
      scrapple

135 - Deer Family
    caribou
    deer (venison)
    elk
    moose
    reindeer

136 - Pronghorn Family
    antelope

137 -   Bovine Family
    beef
    beef by-products
      butter
      cheese
      cow's milk products
        yogurt
      dried milk
      gelatin
      ice cream
      lactose
      oleomargarine
      rennin (rennet)
        sausage
      suet
    veal
    buffalo (bison)
    goat (kid)
      goat's milk
      goat's cheese
      goat's milk yogurt
      sheep (domestic)
        lamb
      mutton
      Rocky Mountain sheep
      Sheep's milk
        Sheep's cheese
          Sheep's yogurt
        Sheep's milk yogurt

* One or more plant parts (leaf, root, seed, etc.) used as beverage.

APPENDIX C

Food & Chemical Effects on Acid / Alkaline Body Chemical Balance

Most Alkaline	More Alkaline	Low Alkaline	Lowest Alkaline	Food Category	Lowest Acid	Low Acid	More Acid	Most Acid
• Baking Soda	Spices/Cinnamon Valerian Licorice • Black Cohash	• Herbs (most) Arnica, Bergamot, Echinacea, Chrysanthemum, Ephedra, Feverfew, Goldenseal, Lemongrass	White Willow Bark Slippery Elm Artemesia Annua	Spice/Herb	Curry	Vanilla Stevia	Nutmeg	Pudding/Jam/Jelly
Sea Salt Mineral Water	• Kambucha	• Green or Mu Tea	*Sulfite* Ginger Tea	Preservative Beverage	*MSG* *Kona Coffee*	*Benzoate* *Alcohol* Black Tea	*Aspartame* *Coffee*	*Table Salt (NaCl)* *Beer; 'Soda'* *Yeast/Hops/Malt*
	Molasses Soy Sauce	Rice Syrup Apple Cider Vinegar	• Sucanat • Umeboshi Vinegar	Sweetener Vinegar	Honey/Maple Syrup Rice Vinegar	*Saccharin* Balsamic Vinegar	*Sugar/Cocoa* *White/Acetic Vinegar*	
• Umeboshi Plum	• Sake		• Algae, Blue-Green	Therapeutic		*Antihistamines*	*Psychotropics*	*Antibiotics*
			• Ghee (Clarified Butter)	Processed Dairy	Cream/Butter	Cow Milk	• Casein, Milk Protein, Cottage Cheese	*Processed Cheese*
			Human Breast Milk	Cow/Human Soy Goat/Sheep	Yogurt Goat/Sheep Cheese	Aged Cheese Soy Cheese Goat Milk	New Cheese Soy Milk	Ice Cream
				Egg	Chicken Egg			
	• Quail Egg		• Duck Egg	Meat Game Fish/Shell Fish Fowl	Gelatin/Organs • Venison Fish Wild Duck	Lamb/Mutton Bear/Elk/Game Meat Shell Fish/Mollusks Goose/Turkey	Pork/Veal Bear • Mussel/Squid Chicken	Beef Lobster • Pheasant
			Oat 'Grain Coffee' • Quinoa Wild Rice Japonica Rice	Grain Cereal Grass	• Triticale Millet Kasha • Amaranth Brown Rice	Buckwheat Wheat • Spelt/Teff/Kamut Farina/Semolina White Rice	Maize Barley Groat Corn Rye Oat Bran	Barley *Processed Flour*
Pumpkin Seed	Poppy Seed Cashew Chestnut Pepper	Primrose Oil Sesame Seed Cod Liver Oil Almond • Sprout	Avocado Oil Seeds (most) Coconut Oil Olive/Macadamia Oil Linseed/Flax Oil	Nut Seed/Sprout Oil	Pumpkin Seed Oil Grape Seed Oil Sunflower Oil Pine Nut Canola Oil	Almond Oil Sesame Oil Safflower Oil Tapioca • Seitan or Tofu	Pistachio Seed Chestnut Oil *Lard* Pecan Palm Kernel Oil	• *Cottonseed Oil/Meal* Hazelnut Walnut Brazil Nut *Fried Food*
Hydrogenated Oil								
Lentil Broccoflower • Seaweed: Nori/Kombu/Wakame/Hijiki Onion/Miso • Daikon/• Taro Root • Sea Vegetables (other) • Burdock/• Lotus Root Sweet Potato/Yam	Kohlrabi Parsnip/Taro Garlic Asparagus Kale/Parsley Endive/Arugula Mustard Greens Ginger Root Broccoli	Potato/Bell Pepper Mushroom/Fungi Cauliflower Cabbage Rutabaga • Salsify/• Ginseng Eggplant Pumpkin Collard Greens	Brussels Sprout Beet Chive/Cilantro Celery/Scallion Okra/Cucumber Turnip Greens Squash Lettuce Jicama	Bean Vegetable Legume Pulse Root	Spinach Fava Bean Kidney Bean Black-eyed Pea String/Wax Bean Zucchini Chutney Rhubarb	Split Pea Pinto Bean White Bean Navy/Red Bean Aduki Bean Lima or Mung Bean Chard	Green Pea Peanut Snow Pea Legumes (other) Carrot Chick Pea/Garbanzo	Soybean Carob
Lime Nectarine Persimmon Raspberry Watermelon Tangerine Pineapple	Grapefruit Cantaloupe Honeydew Citrus Olive • Dewberry Loganberry Mango	Lemon Pear Avocado Apple Blackberry Cherry Peach Papaya	Orange Apricot Banana Blueberry Pineapple Juice Raisin, Currant Grape Strawberry	Citrus Fruit Fruit	Coconut Guava • Pickled Fruit Dry Fruit Fig Persimmon Juice • Cherimoya Date	Plum Prune Tomato	Cranberry Pomegranate	

• Therapeutic, gourmet, or exotic items

Italicized items are NOT recommended

Prepared by Dr. Russell Jaffe, Fellow, Health Studies Collegium. Reprints available from ELISA/ACT Biotechnologies, 14 Pidgeon Hill, #300, Sterling, VA 20165. Sources include USDA food data base (Rev 9 & 10), *Food & Nutrition Encyclopedia*; *Nutrition Applied Personally*, by M. Walczuk; *Acid & Alkaline* by H. Aihara. Food growth, transport, storage, processing, preparation, combination, & assimilation influence effect intensity. Thanks to Hank Liers for his original work. [Rev 10/02]

APPENDIX D
Organizations, Links, Informed References & Sources

ORGANIZATION	Phone	Web	Comments
Beyond Pesticides	202-543-5450	www.beyondpesticides.com	Provides links to useful and related subjects. Printed materials available.
Center for Health, Environment and Justice (CHEJ)	703-237-2249	http://www.chej.org	Founded by Lois Gibbs (Love Canal leader.) Organizes community efforts to hold industry and government accountable.
Chemical Injury Information Network (CIIN)	406-547-2255	http://ciin.org	Non-profit, run by chemically injured for benefit of chemically injured. Outstanding newsletter "Our Toxic Times."
Developmental Delay Resources (DDR)	800-497-0944	www.devdelay.org	Unique newsletter essential for children's health, especially autism spectrum disorders.
Feingold Association	800-321-3287	www.feingold.org	Beginning steps to help children with hyperactivity or "labeled ADHD" & much more.
Human Ecology Study Group	309-685-2437 attention: Vilma		Dedicated to keeping Dr. Randolph's legacy alive. His original support group.
National Vaccine Info Center (NVIC)	703-938-0342	www.nvic.org	Important contact for parents & adults concerned about reactions to vaccines.
New Hope	301-946-6395	www.nhfi.org	Unique program, provides environmentally safe oasis for those with behavioral symptoms.
Well Mind Association Of Greater Washington, D.C.	301-774-6617 attention: Alyce Ortuzar		Holistic medicine information clearing house, focusing on mental health and nutrition. Newsletter identifies treatment options, for informed choices about health.

PROFESSIONAL MEDICAL & DENTAL ORGANIZATIONS				
ORGANIZATION	Phone	Fax	Web	Comments
American Acad. of Environmental Medicine (AAEM)	316-684-5500	316-684-5709	www.aaem.com	Leading group, focusing on environmental causes of illness. Resource for physicians, other health care providers, patients and the public. Closely associated with the American Board of Environmental Medicine, which certifies physicians in the specialty.
American Environmental Health Foundation (AEHF)	800-428-2343	214-361-2534	www.aehf.com	Co-sponsors yearly meetings with AAEM. Profits from catalog sales fund research and symposia.
Int'l Academy of Oral Medicine & Toxicology (IAOMT)	863-420-6373	863-420-6394	www.iaomt.com	Founded in 1984 in Canada, researches physiological effects of dental materials and procedures.
International Society of Orthomolecular Medicine (ISOM)	416-733-2117	416-733-2352	www.orthomed.org	Source and links to programs, centers and journals, optimizing treatments that come from within the body. History of *Journal of Orthomolecular Medicine* by Abram Hoffer is outstanding.
Southwest College of Naturopathic Medicine and Health Sciences	800-858-9100	480-858-0222	www.scnm.edu	Has new Environmental Medicine Center, dedicated to following principles established by Dr. Randolph. Location of Dr. Randolph's library.

PRODUCTS

NO PRODUCT IS SAFE FOR EVERYONE. The following list of sources has been helpful to some of our patients. Try them for starters.

COMPANY	Phone	Fax	Web	Comments
Dust-Free	800-447-1100	800-929-9712	www.dustfree.com	Air purifiers for sensitive individuals. Special inserts available for formaldehyde removal.
Eurosteam	800-613-3874	817-297-6675	www.eurosteam.com	Source for steam cleaning equipment.
Janice Corp	800-526-4237	973-691-5459	www.janices.com	Founded by Janice, an ETI patient. Caution – under new management.
Maggie's Functional Organics	800-609-8593	734-998-1711	www.maggiesorganics.com	Organic cotton clothing and hemp socks. Ask for fabric composition details.
NEEDS	800-631-1380		www.needs.com	Excellent source for relatively safe products and nutrients.
Palmer Industries, Inc.	800-545-8383	301-898-3312		Excellent source for mold remediation and toxic-free sealants.
Sandra DenBraber	817-469-9626	817-860-9299	www.ncchem.com	Source for personalized mask filters.
SMART Air Solutions	800-977-9AIR		SMARTAir@comcast.net	IQAir® Cleaners. Air filters for home, office and mercury removal.

BOOK REFERENCES

Books of Interest – some are cited in the text. Disclaimer: This listing does not imply endorsement of a book's content.

Author	Title	Year	Publisher	Notes
Andrews, Ted	*How to See and Read the Aura*	1999	Llewelyn Publications	For comparison purposes.
Balch, James and Balch, Phyllis	*Prescription for Nutritional Healing*	1998	Avery Publishing Group	Nutrient listings.
Benson, Herbert	*The Relaxation Response*	1975	Avon Books	Early concepts on relaxation.
Colborn, Theo, Dumanoski, Dianne, and Myers, John	*Our Stolen Future*	1996	Dutton	Scientific research that validates the toxic effects on our environment and our need for prevention.
Coyner, Dale	*Motorcycle Journeys through the Appalachians*	1995	White Horse Press	Resource for car vacations in unpolluted areas, phone to check safe lodgings.
Crook, William	*The Yeast Connection*	1989	Professional Books	Resource for identifying yeast problems.
Gerber, Richard	*Vibrational Medicine*	1996	Bear & Co.	Source for understanding energy.
Golos, Natalie and Rea, William J.	*Success in the Clean Bedroom*	1992	Pinnacle Publishers	Foundation for our book. Limited availability. See alanrvinitskymd.com.
Golos, Natalie and Golbitz, Frances Golos	*Coping with Your Allergies*	1986	Fireside Books	Basis for understanding allergic manifestations.
Kilham, Christopher	*The Five Tibetans*	1994	Healing Arts Press	Yoga positioning.

BOOK REFERENCES

Books of Interest – some are cited in the text. Disclaimer: This listing does not imply endorsement of a book's content.

Matthews, Dale A.	*The Faith Factor*	1998	Penguin Books	Spiritual approach to healing.
Mehl-Madrona, Lewis	*Coyote Medicine*	1997	Fireside	Native American approach to healing.
Randolph, Theron G.	*Environmental Medicine – Beginnings & Bibliographies of Clinical Ecology*	1987	Clinical Ecology Publications, Inc.	Extensive reference lists and articles lay a foundation for autonomic neuropathy and environmental analysis.
Randolph, Theron G.	*Human Ecology and Susceptibility to the Chemical Environment*	1962	Charles C. Thomas, Publisher	Early descriptions of environmental illness.
Rapp, Doris J.	*Is This Your Child?*	1991	Morrow	Links behavior change to allergies.
Rapp, Doris J.	*Is This Your Child's World?*	1996	Bantam Books	Further elaboration including evaluation in the school setting.
Rea, William J.	*Chemical Sensitivities*	1992-97	Lewis Press	The acknowledged premier textbook on Chemical Sensitivities.
Redfield, James	*The Celestine Prophecy*	1993	Warner Books	Raises questions about fate and chance.
Sampson, Robert and Hughes, Patricia	*Breaking Out of Environmental Illness*	1997	Bear & Co.	Physician and nurse tell their stories about Chemical Sensitivities.

BOOK REFERENCES

Books of Interest – some are cited in the text. Disclaimer: This listing does not imply endorsement of a book's content.

Author	Title	Year	Publisher	Description
Sears, Barry	*The Zone: A Dietary Road Map*	1995	Harper Collins	Fundamental dietary plan that emphasizes adequate protein and fat.
Sherman, Janette	*Life's Delicate Balance*	2000	Taylor & Francis Group	Identifies causes of breast cancer, evaluates treatment options.
Shoemaker, Ritchie	*Desperation Medicine*	2001	Gateway Press	Identifies neurotoxins as a cause of some illnesses.
Selye, Hans	*The Stress of Life*	1956	McGraw-Hill	One of the first authors writing about the effects of stress on human health.
Varley, Peter editor	*Complementary Therapies in Dental Practice*	1998	Butterworth-Heinemann	Reference for environmental and alternative industry.
Wilson, Duff	*Fateful Harvest*	2001	Harper Collins	Exposé on hazardous materials in the environment.
Wolf, Fred A.	*Eagle's Quest*	1992	Simon & Schuster Trade Paperbacks	Research Ph.D physicist pursues physics of healing in the traditions of shamans, medicine men and more.
Yaron, Ruth	*Super Baby Food*	1998	F.J. Roberts Publishing	Food descriptions and recipes for youngsters.

LINKS OF INTEREST

WEB SITE	WEB ADDRESS	DESCRIPTION
Energy - the Essence of Environmental Health	www. energytheessenceofenvironmentalhealth. com	**Keep your book current!** Read **ALAN'S ACES** and **NATALIE'S NUGGETS** for the latest updates!
ALAN R. VINITSKY, M.D.	www.alanrvinitskymd.com	Information about Dr. Vinitsky's practice, appointments, useful links and more.
NATALIE GOLOS	www.alanrvinitskymd.com	How to find Natalie for personal consultations.

PART X

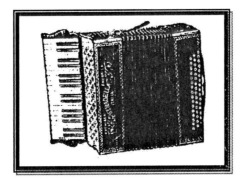

GLOSSARY

GLOSSARY

Accordion Reserve©	Model that depicts your level of health. Describes functional level of your body's energy and the changes of the autonomic nervous system.
ADAPTATION	Adjustment to stress. Prolonged adaptation results in system failure and recognizable medical conditions.
ADDICTION	Craving. Requiring progressively more of a substance of exposure to satisfy symptoms of withdrawal.
ADRENALIN	Neurotransmitter, also called epinephrine, that is a messenger of the sympathetic nervous system.
AURA	Appearance of energy surrounding the physical body.
AUTOMATIC PILOT	Conditioned pattern of relaxation.
AUTONOMIC NERVOUS SYSTEM	Regulator or controller of the body, usually works in the background to regulate and maintain stability.
AUTONOMIC NEUROPATHY	Unbalanced autonomic nervous system.
BELIEF SYSTEM	Your understanding of how and why you exist in the universe.
BINGE	Excessive consumption of a craved substance.
BI-SALTS (SEE TRI-SALTS)	Alkaline preparation that can turn off reactions – sodium and potassium bicarbonates.
Body Awareness	When in a relaxed state, a sense of how your body feels or performs.
BODY TOLERANCE	Level of how much of an exposure can be processed without developing acute or delayed symptoms.
BRAIN FOG	Clouded sensation, inability to think or act with a clear mind.

CHAKRA	Portals for personal energy entry and exit.
CHEMICAL SENSITIVITY	Heightened reactivity to extremely low levels of exposure.
CHI GONG	See Qi Gong.
CHRONIC FATIGUE SYNDROME	Pattern of illness that first was defined by lymph node enlargement and other criteria, but often has autonomic neuropathy as a component.
CILIA	Microscopic beating "hairs" on some cell types, assist in locomotion or transport.
CLINICAL ECOLOGY	Field of medicine, defined by Theron Randolph, M.D., to describe human relationship with his chemical environment. Referred to today as Environmental Medicine.
CONDITIONING	Developing a patterned behavior.
DECONDITIONING	Undoing a patterned behavior.
DETOXICATION	Body's process of handling toxic exposures, mostly in the liver, through a sequence of chemical reactions by converting fat-soluble chemicals into water-soluble for elimination.
DETOXIFICATION	Treatment protocol to improve detoxication.
DETOXIFY	Clear a toxin from the body.
DISTILLED WATER	Purified water that was collected after boiling at 212°.
DISTRESS	A negative energy (undesirable) stress that results in a shrinking **Accordion Reserve**©.
ELECTROMAGNETIC FIELD (EMF)	Energy field generated by electron motion.
ELIMINATION DIET	General term for removing potentially allergic foods from the diet on a trial basis.
ELIMINATION TEST	Avoidance of exposure, observing for symptoms worsening during first 4 days, improving over next 3 days and recurrent symptoms on rechallenge.
ENDORPHINS	Chemical mediators that have a "feel-good" effect on behavior, symptoms and well-being.

ENVIRONMENTAL HEALTH   State of well-being, resulting from applying the principles of the *Accordion Reserve*©.

ENVIRONMENTAL MEDICINE   Field of medicine that addresses the effects of environmental (biologic, chemical and physical) influences on human health.

ENVIRONMENTALLY TRIGGERED ILLNESS   Conditions that are more likely to be associated with or caused by biological, chemical or physical exposures.

EUSTRESS   Positive (desirable) stress that results in an enlarging *Accordion Reserve*©.

Exercise Sandwich©   Behavioral pattern of dividing a meal into 2 parts and inserting movement (exercise) between the parts.

FAITH HEALING   The practice or art of utilizing meditation, relaxation and *Soul Searching*, in the context of a belief system to promote healing.

FIBROMYALGIA   Defined by tender trigger points in at least 11 of 18 muscle sites. Frequently associated with or caused by autonomic neuropathy.

FOG HEAD   Our new expression to describe individuals with "brain fog."

FORMALDEHYDE   Volatile chemical, that offgases from plywood, particleboard, some insulation foams, wrinkle-free clothing, etc.

FUMES   Undesirable gases emitted from solvents, paints, gasoline and others.

GIARDIA   Parasite that sometimes causes symptoms like milk intolerance — gas, diarrhea and bloating.

GROUND REGULATING SYSTEM   Channel between blood vessels and cells that allows for complex interactions of nerves, hormones and inflammatory messengers. Location of some acupuncture meridians.

GROUNDED   State of balanced relaxation that allows for sensing *Body Awareness*.

343

GROUNDING	Process of balancing energy flow during **Meditation/Relaxation**.
GULF WAR SYNDROME	Complex pattern of illnesses that share features with autonomic neuropathy, chronic fatigue, chemical sensitivity, fibromyalgia and post-traumatic stress disorder.
HEAT EXHAUSTION	Early stage of body overheating, identified by gooseflesh, shivers and feeling cold, in a heated environment.
HEAT STROKE	Late stage, life-threatening body overheating, accompanied by mental deterioration and other severe neurologic symptoms.
HERBICIDES	Pesticides that are used to kill or poison undesirable plant growth.
HISTAMINE	A chemical mediator most often linked with allergy. Its depletion in whole blood is often associated with an overactive sympathetic nervous system.
HOLOGRAM	A three-dimensional image created by intersecting laser beams. May be sensed during **Meditation/Relaxation**.
HOMOCYSTEINE	Transitional amino acid, made from methionine, which is inflammatory and is linked to vascular disease.
HYPOTHALAMIC-PITUITARY AXIS	Connection and pathways in the deeper sections of the brain, linked to the autonomic nervous system.
IDEOMOTOR	Conditioned learned behavior that resembles a response from a trigger.
INSECTICIDES	Pesticides that are used to rid an environment of specific insects.
INTEGRATED PEST MANAGEMENT	Progressive planning program to control pests without harming desirable aspects of environment and human population.
LABILE HYPERTENSION	Fluctuating elevations of blood pressure that vary in a short time period.
MAGNETIC	Sense of feeling "opposites" attract and "likes" repel.

MASKING	Gradually reduced symptoms, even as the exposure continues, causing a reduced **Accordion Reserve**©.
Meditation/Relaxation Healing	Using parasympathetic nervous system breathing to induce relaxation and eventually healing.
MERIDIANS	Pathways that course the body in the ground regulating system and other locations.
Mind/body/soul/spirit	Unification of all parts of a living human, maximizing energy potential, promoting environmental health and expanded energy.
MOLD	General term for a group of organisms that include fungi and yeast. Affects humans by producing chemicals like hexane and neurotoxins. Promotes allergy. Toxins they produce are the basis for antibiotics.
NEGATIVE THINKING	Adverse impact on your **Accordion Reserve**©. A form of distress.
NEUROTRANSMITTER	Chemical mediator that affects nervous system function.
NITROSAMINE	Potent carcinogen, which was used as a food additive. Found in rubberized materials. Made in the stomach, when exposed to nitrite. Inhibited by ascorbate (vitamin C).
NUCLEUS SOLITARIUS	Site in the brain stem where an excessively dominant sympathetic nervous system can suppress the parasympathetic.
OASIS	Safe place to encourage healing. Requirements: relatively clean air, food and water, nutrients, effective sleep, exercise and relationships.
OFFGAS	Emit odor or "odor-free" vapors from a material. Examples: paint, even after the paint is dry; appliances constructed from plastic.
OLFACTORY CHALLENGE	Stimulus for the sense of smell. Olfactory nerve connects to brain region (limbic system) that responds quickly with a stress response.

OLFACTORY FATIGUE	Stimulus is turned off quickly. Warning is then ignored. "Getting used to the smell." Like adaptation, has long-term adverse consequences.
ORGANIC FOOD	Certified, grown in the absence of pesticides, antibiotics and hormones. Varies by state regulation. Undermining the certification: after production handling, transporting and co-mingling non-organic products that contaminate.
ORTHOSTATIC	Postural, as in changing from sitting to standing.
OZONE	Three oxygen atoms in one molecule. Potent oxidizing agent. Can be harnessed to sometimes help clear a site of contamination.
PARASYMPATHETIC	Healing and energy-conserving branch of the autonomic nervous system.
PESTICIDE	Composite term for insecticides, herbicides, fungicides, rodenticides and others. Used to get rid of pests of any kind.
Playing with Your Aura©	Using sensed personal energy to promote healing.
POSITIVE THINKING	Applying energy in a useful way to expand the **Accordion Reserve©**.
PRESERVATIVE	Substance that prolongs the existence of another substance. May be natural or synthetic.
PSEUDOMONAS	Type of Gram-negative usually anaerobic bacteria that most often cause urine or other infections.
QI GONG	(pronounced "chi") System of personal energy management and balance in Eastern Medicine.
RECONDITIONING	Re-establishing or revising a habit or learned behavior.
REINFORCEMENT	Influence on the outcome of a conditioned behavior. Comes in 3 "flavors" — positive, negative and intermittent.

SEROTONIN	Neurotransmitter for calming and sleep generation. Derived from tryptophan.
SERENDIPITY	"Chance" occurrence. Central phenomenon to the debate on fate, destiny and choice in life's experience.
SHIELDING	Protection, insulation, isolating or providing safety to Mind/body/soul/spirit.
SHORTCUT	Personally conditioned behavior that quickly induces Meditation/Relaxation breathing.
SNIFF TEST	Using Body Awareness as a detective. Technique to identify potential adverse responses to exposures.
SOLVENT	Liquid in which a substance can be dissolved. As in the phrase "petroleum-based" solvent, a carrier for an active ingredient, such as a pesticide. Very toxic, yet is labeled "inert" or "inactive."
SPIRITUAL GUIDANCE	Assistance from a spiritual aide during a Soul Searching experience.
SPIRITUAL HEALING	Resulting from practiced behaviors of Meditation/Relaxation, Body Awareness, grounding, balancing the autonomic nervous system and Soul Searching. Influenced by your Guiding Force and belief system.
SWIVEL MANEUVER	Technique for enhancing visualization of your aura.
SYMPATHETIC	"Fright, then flight or fight" stress response of the autonomic nervous system.
SYNCHRONICITY	Moving along a parallel or similar path over time. While parallel lines never cross, serendipitous events permit paths to intersect, introduce shifts of awareness and alter future events.
T'AI-CHI	System of energy management in Eastern Medicine.
TARGET PRACTICE	Three-step conditioning technique for potty training.

TERRIBLE TWO'S	Toddler age mislabeled for the apparent misbehavior of children. "Bad behavior" should be respected and handled as a message to teach children to handle emotions safely.
The Awakening	Insight to your sense of personal Meditation/Relaxation.
TOURETTE'S SYNDROME	Motor and vocal disorder of uncontrollable and unpredictable tics, often of genetic origin, and influenced by environmental, nutritional and energy factors.
TOXIC ENCEPHALOPATHY	Dysfunction of brain tissue, resulting from environmental insult.
TOXIN	Substance that adversely affects function. Classically, more than a certain minimum dose produces a greater effect. Newer thinking demonstrates that minimal doses may have a magnified effect.
TRI-SALTS	Alkaline preparation to turn off reactions — sodium and potassium bicarbonates and calcium carbonate. Magnesium can be substituted for sodium.
TRYPTOPHAN	Amino acid precursor for serotonin and niacin.
VAGUS NERVE	Major nerve that carries parasympathetic messages from brain stem to organs.
VALUE SYSTEM	A set of personal standards that are the basis for decision making.
VASCULITIS	Inflammation of blood vessels. Basis for many multi-organ system illnesses because blood vessels supply all organs.
VIBRATION	State of energy movement. Depends on electron motion in atoms and molecules.
VISUALIZATION	Technique of sensing an image that promotes a change in your energy state.
VOLATILE ORGANIC COMPOUNDS	Chemicals derived from carbon skeletons that exist mostly as liquid but become a vapor at usual ambient temperatures.

WHITE COAT
HYPERTENSION

High blood pressure readings recorded in a doctor's office.

WITHDRAWAL

Absence of a substance of exposure results in symptoms.

YOGA

General term to describe methods of relaxation and stretching of muscles.

PART XI

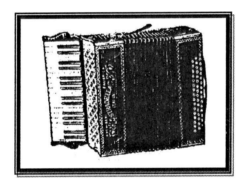

INDEX

INDEX

ABOUT THE AUTHORS

Based on her personal experiences with Environmentally Triggered Illness Natalie Golos has written 6 books, notably the internationally acclaimed *Coping with Your Allergies, If It's Tuesday, it must be Chicken,* and *Success in the Clean Bedroom.* In addition to her experience as an English teacher, she has logged more than 9 years of study in Bio-energy Therapies and 2000 hours of Continuing Medical Education in Environmental Medicine, preventive medicine, orthomolecular medicine, functional medicine and nutrition.

Alan R. Vinitsky, M.D. is a successful primary care physician who broadened his interests in Environmental Medicine after meeting Natalie at a local medical grand rounds. He received his medical degree from the University of Pennsylvania School of Medicine, completed residencies in Internal Medicine at Upstate Medical Center, Syracuse and Pediatrics at Children's Hospital of Philadelphia. Board-certified in both specialties, he continued studies and passed exams in the field of Environmental Medicine. Alan has long been interested in teaching patients, parents and children creative ways to improve their health. Self-trained as a marathon runner, Alan gained valuable expertise and insight from the power of listening to his body.

Together Natalie and Alan turned their unique talents into a collaboration of adventure and discovery. Join them on the road to healing and recovery, as they unravel the mystery of achieving optimal health.

Printed in the United States
22499LVS00004B/40-279